Stop the Clock

The Optimal Anti-Aging Strategy

P. D. Mangan

Phalanx Press

Contents

Introduction

A strategy to slow or reverse aging already exists

In this book, we'll discuss the best strategy that is currently available for slowing and even reversing the aging process. This strategy requires nothing expensive – in fact, if so inclined, you could implement it at no cost whatsoever.

The strategy, while in theory and in practice is simple enough, is backed solidly by science. No wild claims will be made here, and no sales pitches made for some kind of magic potion or hormone that will cure all your ills and make you live to 120, because no such potion exists.

Humans have been concerned with preventing or slowing down aging ever since they understood what it means to get old. From the quest for the Fountain of Youth to modern-day quack treatments, men stumbled their way trying to find something, anything, that would restore to them a measure of youth. In the first years of the 16th century, one man, Luigi Cornaro, made a major discovery in anti-aging medicine, and although he applied his discovery successfully to his own life, lengthening it to over 100 years, he lacked the means to understand its mechanism of action. More major discoveries had to wait until the 20th century, when the science of biology had advanced enough that scientists could make sense of their results and to expand on them.

The science of aging in the 21st century is now in full bloom, with literally dozens of scientific journals devoted exclusively to that topic, and thousands of scientists working on the problem of aging. Those scientists are making real progress, and we can now say that we possess fundamental knowledge of the causes of aging as well as the knowledge of various techniques and substances that have the ability to retard aging. Scientific journals publish new advances in the science of aging daily.

This is not to say that the problems of aging have been solved, not by a long shot. But we can now quite accurately describe many of the processes that occur during aging, and with this ability comes the opportunity and maybe the ability to counteract them. What is more, many of the substances and processes that can counteract aging can be easily obtained or practiced by almost everyone. No expensive anti-aging clinics and no expensive drugs are required. Anyone who has the interest and a bit of discipline can make available to themselves nearly everything science currently knows about retarding the aging process.

Aging as it is properly understood begins when a person is in his or her twenties. Already by the decade of the late twenties, brainpower begins to decline. By the decade of the thirties, muscle mass and strength are noticeably lower in both men and women. This fact explains why many professional athletes retire when in their late twenties or early thirties: their bodies are aged in terms of elite athletics, even though they're chronologically young, and they can't keep up with the younger athletes, who are in their prime, which is their teens and twenties. The process of aging at what we consider a relatively youthful age is merely more noticeable in athletes, since they must be on top of their game, but it happens to everyone. *The point is that it's never too early to do something about aging.* It shouldn't be a concern of only the elderly, who would like to prolong their lives and prevent and cure disease, but of virtually all adults, in order to live full of strength and vitality and to extend the time that they are able to live healthy, active lives.

Fighting aging and living a longer life does not mean extending the time in which we are old and frail and living in a nursing home, which is a common objection to the idea of life extension. *The purpose of fighting aging is to remain in a youthful, vital state, free of disease and illness, as long as possible.* Ideally, life extension means that "old age" should be a period in our lives when we can remain in a youthful state as much as possible, and any decline in function or susceptibility to disease will be confined to a period very shortly before death.

Personally, I am not looking for an extension of decades in which I need to use a cane, or a walker, or an oxygen tank, or powerful drugs with huge unwanted side effects, and the reader undoubtedly is not either. What I am looking for is many decades in which I do not need these things.

For the elderly, aging can take on a tragic aspect, with the specter of diseases like Alzheimer's and Parkinson's, sarcopenia (muscle wasting), diabetes, heart disease, and cancer. Many of the elderly become so frail that they become unable to take care of themselves, and end up in nursing homes. Many of these problems can be entirely avoided if the right steps are taken, and some of them can be fixed even in the very old.

While it's never too early to start taking steps to fight aging, in many cases it's never too late either.

Even people that are considered young are not immune to the ravages of age. How many middle-aged men and women have we seen that suffer from obesity, diabetes and metabolic syndrome, who do not sleep well, suffer from anxiety and depression, and in general have little vitality and do not enjoy the energy and vitality that is theirs by birthright? A rhetorical question. All of these ailments increase dramatically with age, that is, they are symptoms of aging.

A lifestyle that incorporates the anti-aging practices discussed in this book need not be either expensive or time-consuming, but it will, as I say, take a bit of discipline. The world tempts us with obesogenic food, a passive and inactive way of life, a desire for a quick fix for everything that ails us, and conspires to lure us into its pro-aging ways. Make no mistake, *if you do what almost everyone around you is doing, you will age just as fast as they do*, buoyed only by the hope that some new drug will save you from a debilitating disease of old age.

To fight aging, you must resist the siren songs of the pro-aging environment which is everywhere around us.

Actuarial Escape Velocity

The concept of actuarial escape velocity has been championed by the theorist of aging Aubrey de Grey, and by the futurist Ray Kurzweil. The idea is that science and medicine have been able to increase the human lifespan year after year, and that the rate at which they do this is itself increasing. As a hypothetical example, ten years from now, scientific advances may have been able to increase the average human lifespan by five years; but in the next ten year span, it may have increased average lifespan by eight years. Eventually a point comes such that for each year of scientific research, average lifespan will go up by more than one year, and at that point actuarial escape velocity will have been reached. At that point, and assuming that the rate of scientific advance at least remains the same, the average person could expect to live indefinitely, if of course they have access to the advances that have been made, and other events don't intercede, such as wars, accidents, or homicides.

From a logical point of view, it looks like actuarial escape velocity is all but inevitable, unless there is something about aging and absolute limits that exists but that we do not currently understand, or if the current rate of technological and scientific advance slows for some reason.

However, to see the day that actuarial escape velocity becomes a reality, we must do what is in our power to avoid and retard aging now. Most people would likely be surprised to learn just how much is possible in this area. Many of the techniques and compounds that slow or reverse aging are the same as those that keep us in good general health. Exercise is an example of this. It's been said that if exercise were a pill, it would be the most widely prescribed medicine there is. Exercise can prevent and even cure diabetes, heart disease, cancer, dementia, and a host of other diseases and symptoms of aging.

Median versus maximum lifespan

Exercise is, however, an example of something that increases median lifespan, but not maximum lifespan.

What's the difference between median and maximum lifespan? When scientists study a substance or process that may extend lifespan, they distinguish between the two. Take the example of exercise. If one group of animals is exercised, or allowed to exercise, while another group of animals (the "controls") remain or are kept sedentary, more of the exercising animals will live into old age than the sedentary; but the absolute, or maximum, lifespan of the two groups will remain the same. Exercise increases median lifespan.

If a substance or process causes a large fraction of the test group to live longer lives than the controls, then that substance or process extends maximum lifespan.

Greater median lifespan means that some form of illness or disease that reduces lifespan has been overcome. But other aging processes then come to the fore, and the absolute lifespan remains the same.

An increase in maximum lifespan means that aging itself has been slowed. So, while incorporating practices that lead to good health generally will conduce to an increase in median lifespan, they will not increase maximum lifespan.

Good health practices such as a decent diet or a good exercise regimen will help increase or median lifespan, that is, they will help us reach our full life expectancy. These are absolutely necessary in the fight against aging. There are other processes and compounds that do more than keep us in good health, however; they can go beyond this and slow or reverse aging. An example of a process that can do this is fasting in any of its many variations. Intermittent or alternate day fasting mimics the process of calorie restriction, which has been shown to be the most robust anti-aging treatment known to date. This is where some discipline comes into play, since if you feel the need to eat every three hours, you can't fast and you will not have available the option of fasting in order to intervene in the aging process. Certain well-known, safe, and cheap chemical compounds can mimic the effects of calorie restriction and fasting, compounds such as resveratrol and curcumin.

In this book, we'll discuss these processes and compounds, as well as the optimal anti-aging strategy, so that those who put these into practice will have the best chance possible of reaching the time of actuarial escape velocity. But they must be put into practice; merely reading about them will do nothing.

Chapter 1: Couch Potatoes vs. Hormesis

We've all heard the term "couch potato", referring to someone who takes things easy at all times. The term conjures up the image of an overweight person, lying on the couch with a TV remote in his hands, eating from a bag of potato chips, never bothering to get up if he (usually it's a he) can possibly help it. The couch potato puts himself (or of course, herself) at serious risk for the diseases of modern life, which include heart disease, cancer, diabetes, depression, arthritis, and if he's old enough, osteoporosis and dementia, to name a few. Intuitively we know that the couch potato does virtually everything wrong from the standpoint of health, without knowing exactly why that is. So let me explain.

Humans evolved in an environment of physiological stress

Humans evolved in an environment in which various physiological stresses were a fact of everyday life. In fact, if we go back further, to a time before humans, we see that all of life evolved that way. Competition from the members of the same species, as well as predation from members of other species, has always been endemic for all living things. Humans have always been subject to periods of time in which they've had little to eat. This doesn't mean that they endured constant famines or the threat of them, and in fact, recent research has uncovered the fact that hunter-gatherer peoples have faced famine less often than agricultural peoples.[1] However, humans were hunter-gatherers for about 99% of the time that they've existed as humans, only 1% of the time have they lived as farmers and herders, and even less time still have they lived in an industrial age with cheap and plentiful food, so we can profit from the point of view of health by paying attention to how the hunter-gatherers lived.

Hunter-gatherers did not endure famine as much as did agriculturalists, but they did face having to hunt and gather their food on a daily basis, and thus they could not eat until these tasks had been completed. Given the near total absence of any means of preserving food such as refrigeration or canning, *most humans throughout history just could not eat whenever they felt hungry*, unlike today. Those humans would likely have experienced near daily periods of many hours in which they didn't eat. Among many hunter-gatherer groups that have been studied, it appears that the usual practice was to spend the day in food collecting activities, and then to have a huge meal toward the end of the day when all the food was ready to be cooked and eaten. To compare ourselves with them, it might be good to ask yourself *when was the last time you went without food for twenty-four hours, or even sixteen hours. For the vast majority of people in the modern world, the answer is "never"*. Compared to our ancestors of long ago, we are practically all couch potatoes. We eat whenever we feel like it, which is a privilege that few humans in history could have even dreamed of. Yet it affects our health in ways that few understand.

We evolved in a rugged environment, and that is what we're adapted to. Our environment now is luxurious by comparison, and we are not adapted to that. Hence, the "diseases of civilization".

The evolution of human beings in this rugged environment means that our genes have been selected to be optimal for going relatively long periods, say from twelve to twenty four hours or even longer, without food. When we then switch environments to one in which food is plentifully and readily available at any time of day or night, our genes go awry and lead us into ill health, such as diabetes, and worse.[2] We are not cut out to be couch potatoes; good health and long life requires that our bodies be subject to stresses of various kinds, one such stress being regular periods of refraining from eating. These stresses were a regular part of human life for 99% of our history, and we are adapted to them.

The concept of hormesis

Going without food for a dozen or more hours at a stretch indeed places a stress on the body, a good kind that has been called eustress, but which modern science refers to as hormesis. Hormesis means simply to the placing of a stress on a living organism that the organism is able to respond to and recover from by becoming stronger. Think of it in Nietzschean terms: what doesn't kill you makes you stronger (though of course that's an exaggeration not meant to be taken literally).

Paracelsus (1493-1541), the Renaissance physician and alchemist and founder of the discipline of toxicology, first enunciated the principle that "the dose makes the poison". This expression refers to the fact that any substance at all, even water, can be poisonous in the right dose. But it also follows from this that some substances that we normally think of as poisons are not toxic in low doses, and in fact some of these putative poisons can be healthful for the human body if taken in the right amount. They do this by placing a stress on the body, and on each of the cells in it, and by doing so strengthen the body.

The process of going without food, that is, fasting, is an example of hormesis, although in this case it is not a chemical substance that places the stress, but the absence of nutrients from food. With fasting, as with other forms of hormesis, the dose makes the poison. Fasting for long periods of time can lead to weakness, a declining immune system, and ultimately death. But in low doses, fasting places a hormetic stress on the body, which then strengthens itself to deal with the stress.

The concept of hormesis has broad applicability to a wide range of practices, processes, and substances that humans are exposed to, or in the case of many modern humans, not exposed to. *It might even be said that hormesis is the key to health, for without regular applications of hormetic substances and processes, the body cannot remain healthy*. We'll see shortly how hormesis is one leg of our anti-aging regimen. The key to the effect of hormesis is that we have evolved with genes that *expect* stresses, and our health suffers when we are not exposed to them. Since health is so intimately linked with aging, *in order to retard the aging process, we must expose ourselves regularly to healthy hormetic stresses*.

Hormesis can result from low-dose exposure to anything, or any process, that in larger doses is toxic. When a substance or process is toxic, this means that it causes damage to the body and to its cells, damage which causes illness and from which recovery may be difficult or impossible, and in the most extreme cases leads to death. In hormesis, low-doses of the same substance or process signal the body that it must prepare itself for defense, and it does this by various means.

Exercise is an example of hormesis.[3] When a human or animal exercises enough to go beyond its normal limits of adaptation, cells generate reactive oxygen species (ROS), which are more familiarly known as free radicals. These ROS act as signaling molecules which tell the cells to increase their production of antioxidant defenses, DNA repair enzymes, and muscle protein synthesis. In this way, cells and organs thus strengthen themselves in response to a low-dose of a toxin, in this case free radicals, and the person who exercises ends up healthier and stronger than before. This is classic hormesis. Yet, recall the story of the first marathon runner, Phillipides: he ran much farther than what he was trained for, and died. His exercise went beyond the capabilities of his body and was therefore extremely toxic for him.

The free radical theory of aging holds that aging occurs because free radicals cause the accumulation of damage, and therefore the body becomes unable to function as well as it did in the youthful state, much like an automobile runs worse as it gets older, and is more subject to breakdown.[4] While this theory has its merits, it's lately become less compelling as a description of what really happens in aging. One reason for this is the phenomenon of free radical hormesis, which causes damage, as in the case of exercise, yet leaves the organism in a more youthful state than before. *Damage is an intrinsic part of the exercise process, yet there's universal agreement among medical scientists that exercise is among the most healthful things that anyone can undertake.* If exercise were a drug, it would be the most widely prescribed one in the world.

So there's a paradox here: hormesis causes damage, yet it leaves the organism better off, more youthful, than before. Therefore, it seems, the cause of aging cannot be the accumulation of damage, since hormesis would then *increase* aging, when in fact it *decreases* it.

Consider other cases of hormesis, for example, the unusual case of arsenite, a molecule that contains an arsenic atom and that's one of the most toxic substances known to man. (Don't worry, this book will not be advocating the ingestion of arsenite.) Arsenite has been linked to a number of diseases, including heart disease, diabetes, and cancer; yet it was also used in traditional Chinese medicine, and a 1% solution of sodium arsenite, known as Fowler's solution, was in general medical use for the treatment of parasitic infections and other indications until the 1950s. When mammalian (human and mouse) cells are cultured with low doses of arsenite, *their growth is increased*, and when the model organism *C. elegans*, a worm, is raised with arsenite as part of its growth medium, *it increases its lifespan*[5].

What's happening here? Well, it appears that arsenite causes a transient increase in those damaging free radicals, and the cells then upgrade their internal, biochemical stress mechanisms in order to deal with them. One of the more potent mechanisms, which is known as Nrf-2, is a gene transcription factor, which causes the activation of many different genes, most of them related to stress defense. (Later in this book, we'll see how other factors that are more commonly encountered than arsenite also increase Nrf-2, and how this leads to better health and retards aging.) Basically, this means that causing damage through an increase in free radicals ultimately results in less damage and less aging.

Evolutionarily conserved mechanisms

These results are also important because they show *an evolutionarily conserved mechanism*. This means that natural selection chose the means of dealing with abundant free radicals by upgrading cellular stress defenses a long time ago, in primitive organisms, and that through the course of evolution, higher organisms including mammals and humans have retained the ability to do so. Eukaryotic cells, that is, the cells of all organisms further along in evolution than bacteria, share fundamental similarities, and this is one of them. This can be seen in the fact that the same chemical, arsenite, both extended lifespan in a small worm and caused mammalian cells in culture to grow better. Keep this in mind as we extend this discussion throughout the book, as many of the studies and experiments that will I will use as illustrative were done on non-human animals and cell cultures. A common objection to these types of studies is that they do not necessarily translate into what is good for humans; while there's some truth in that objection, and we must carefully consider each study in detail to determine whether it has validity for human beings, the main point of performing studies on non-human animals and cell cultures is because we can find out things that we never could if only humans were used. For example, it would be unethical to give arsenite to humans, but it's acceptable to feed it to a worm. Similarly, scientists can't force humans to swim until they can't hold themselves above water, something that they do with mice. In this book, I will be citing a number of animal and cell culture studies, and except where noted, I consider them to have validity for human beings.

Hormesis is characterized by a so-called U-shaped curve, usually depicted upside down. This can be seen in the following graph, generalizable to all kinds of hormetic responses. It can be seen that a very low or zero dose of a hormetic agent or process, in this particular case exercise, does not create good health, but that as the dose increases, the organism that exercises moves into the zone of good health. At some dose of exercise, the organism reaches optimal health, and at higher doses, movement away from the optimal dose occurs, until a point is reached at which the dose is too high, and ill health or even death occurs.

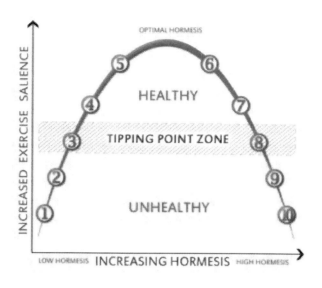

To use a more concrete example, the couch potato who does no exercise lives around point number 1 in the graph. If he starts to exercise even a little, he will rapidly move up the hormetic curve toward the healthy zone, at say point 3 or 4. Someone who exercises the right amount, about which we'll speculate later, lives in the optimal zone, between points 5 and 6. Someone who exercises too much, and in my opinion elite marathon runners may fall into this category, tips into the unhealthy zone, at points 8 through 10.

What evidence is there that hormesis can retard aging? Studies like the one cited above concerning arsenite show that small doses of toxins extend lifespan in laboratory animals and cause human cultured cells to grow better, which is the very definition of hormesis. One study showed that injecting duck eggs with small doses of methylmercury, an extremely toxic compound, or feeding low doses of it to female ducks, led to a hatching success rate of 93%, as opposed to one for controls not fed methylmercury of 73%. [7] In this case, low doses of a toxin led to lower mortality.

Low-dose radiation is another example of hormesis.[8] Low doses of radiation have been shown to decrease the incidence of cancer in mice by more than half.[9] Exposure to solar radiation is negatively associated with the incidence of breast cancer and colon cancer [10], which is another way of saying that the more exposure to the sun people get, within reason, the fewer the number of them that come down with breast or colon cancer, or indeed, other types of cancer. While some of the effect of solar radiation may be due to its interaction with the skin in the production of vitamin D, the effect of the actual ionizing radiation from the sun likely has its own effect on reducing cancer rates. Perhaps the most amazing example of exposure to radiation leading to lower cancer rates occurred in Taiwan, where apartment buildings were constructed with steel that was contaminated with cobalt-60, a radioactive isotope. Up to 10,000 people were unwittingly exposed to ionizing radiation in these apartments for periods of up to several years. A study that looked at these people found dramatically reduced rates of both cancer and congenital malformations.[11]

Older people including centenarians who are in good health often have high levels of the important internal antioxidant glutathione. This is significant for hormesis and aging because hormetic agents frequently result in an increase in glutathione levels, thus demonstrating that hormesis can result in good health and longer life.[12] In aging, levels of the enzymes that increase glutathione levels decline, but healthier elderly people have higher levels than the non-healthy. The increase in glutathione levels through substances and processes that cause hormesis is one of the most important of their health-producing and anti-aging effects, one that we'll look at in more detail later.

In contrast, lack of hormesis results in accelerated aging. Diabetes is perhaps the archetype of aging, with increased insulin resistance, increased inflammation and oxidative stress, fat gain, muscle loss, and increased susceptibilities to all of the diseases of aging, including cancer, heart disease, and infections. Diabetes (type 2) is also basically a lifestyle disease, caused by lack of exercise, weight gain, and eating too much dietary carbohydrate, along with genetic susceptibility. Hormetic factors such as exercise, fasting, and dietary phytochemicals such as those in fruits and vegetables and certain supplements defend against the development of diabetes, and at least in some cases can lead to a complete cure.[13,14] Low-carbohydrate diets should be considered the first line of treatment in diabetes [15], and since diabetes is the archetype of aging, this has implications for life extension as well, which we'll discuss later. In practicing an anti-aging lifestyle, we should avoid as much as possible all those things that lead to diabetes, and to remain in a state opposed to that: lean, with good insulin sensitivity and with low levels of inflammation and oxidative stress, as this state is the anti-aging phenotype.

Hormetic stresses lead to better health and longer life, whether in laboratory animals or in humans. The couch potato life leads to accelerated aging, greater mortality, more illness, and much less vitality.

Most health-conscious people are likely to encounter three main forms of hormesis in their everyday life: exercise, dietary phytochemicals, and fasting. Health experts have of course recommended exercise since the days of Hippocrates, and most people know that eating your fruits and vegetables, the source of most dietary phytochemicals, is also a healthy thing to do. Fasting hasn't received much notice until relatively recently, that is, outside of fairly fringe health movements, but its potential is quite real, and easy-to-do methods of fasting can be incorporated into the routine of anyone interested in slowing the aging process. The next three chapters in the book will discuss each of these three anti-aging modalities in some detail.

The old expression "use it or lose it" finds new meaning in the process of hormesis, or good stress. Muscles atrophy if we don't place regular stress on them, as do our brains, our bones, and virtually every other part of our bodies. Exercise can be thought of as the prototype of good stress or hormesis, since each type of hormesis, whether a chemical compound or a physical activity, essentially causes the cellular systems of our bodies to experience a workout, the physiological equivalent of a hard session at the gym. From these, the cellular systems emerge stronger, ready to defend themselves from outside toxins and foreign invaders such as pathogenic bacteria and viruses, and from internal stresses, resulting in lower levels of inflammation and oxidative stress.

One of the keys to aging lies in the old wisdom to never let yourself go and to stay in good shape. It might almost be said that much of the advice to live a long, healthy life can be boiled down to two words: avoid comfort, at least most of the time. Aging must be combated pro-actively, since it is an all-but-inexorable force that will succeed if we don't fight back. This requires some discipline, though not necessarily an iron will, since the benefits of anti-aging compounds and processes become apparent relatively soon in the form of good health and abundant energy, not merely in retarding aging. Most people will find the program I outline in this book to be enjoyable, or at least, not too difficult; in any case, I enjoy them, and the results in terms of increased physical energy, mental clarity, and good mood make me very much inclined to continue doing them.

Fighting the aging process is much like keeping a building in good repair: the old must be swept out to make way for the new, and maintenance must be made a priority. When we fail to maintain the roof of our house, or let it go without new paint, sooner or later the house will become a decrepit mess, falling apart at the seams and at some point no longer fit to live in. So with our bodies, except that our bodies have the advantage over a house in that if we give them what they need, they will do the repair and maintenance themselves.

Indiscipline, as manifested in eating too much, or too much of the wrong kind of food, or as we'll see, too often, as well as failure to exercise, results in accelerated aging and the diseases of age, such as heart disease, cancer, and diabetes. The couch potato lifestyle in which one indulges oneself with modern, industrial foods and the complacencies of the peignoir (to quote Wallace Stevens) or, as we might say, the comforts of the sofa, allows the aging process full reign. Fighting aging doesn't at all mean that the pleasures of life must be avoided, although depending on your definition of pleasure, some of them certainly will. (I like a good glass of wine as much as the next person, and fortunately wine in moderation turns out to be one of the healthy pleasures.) But it does mean that attention must be paid, that some part of every day must be devoted to ensuring that you have all of your anti-aging ducks in a row.

The Three Processes Involved in Aging

Aging correlates most notably with an increase in the susceptibility to illness and disease, which is practically the definition of aging. Getting older almost always equates with being in a state of worse health: minor illnesses like colds are easier to get and harder to overcome, while infections such as the flu that cause transient illness in younger people have the potential to kill the elderly. Diseases resulting from a breakdown of the body's structure range from arthritis to dementia and increase greatly with aging. Strokes, heart disease, cancer: they all come from a fundamental inability of the aging body to properly maintain and repair itself. Therefore, to fight aging, we must do those things that allow the body to keep its maintenance and repair capabilities.

Why does aging cause the loss of these capabilities? Younger people have a far greater ability to defend their bodies against infection and to maintain the body's normal, youthful structure. *Aging means a breaking down of capacity for renewal.* Something occurs as we age that hinders that capacity.

Three main processes are responsible for the deterioration of aging: 1) an increase in oxidative stress; 2) an increase in inflammation; and 3) a decline in autophagy, or the process of ridding cells of junk in order to replace it with new, more functional structures. They are all closely linked, and in most cases improvement in one of these processes entails improvement in the others.

Oxidative stress refers to the inability of cells to maintain a proper balance of free radicals. As we've mentioned, free radicals (or reactive oxygen species, ROS) function as signaling molecules, but too many of them cause damage that cannot be repaired. The body must balance the amount of free radicals present: not too few, not too many. As we age, that balance becomes more difficult to attain, and free radicals overwhelm the body's internal antioxidant system; when that happens, a state of oxidative stress exists. In oxidative stress, free radicals have free reign inside cells, and cause damage to cellular structures, meaning that these structures will no longer function as well as in a youthful state. If we consider the case of infections, which afflict the elderly harder and more often than they do the young, the reason is that the immune system doesn't function as well in the elderly, so it can't fight infections effectively. The immune cells have been damaged by oxidative stress among other things.

In the inflammation of aging, the immune system is activated consistently but at a low level. This is such a strong characteristic of aging that it has been dubbed "inflammaging".[6] The cause of inflammaging appears to be lifelong exposure to various infectious agents, against which the immune system mounts a response. This results in a chronic, low level of inflammation that contributes to illness and death from old age. Healthy centenarians appear to have a higher level of anti-inflammatory compounds, called cytokines, that balance and counteract inflammatory cytokines. As we get older, inflammaging causes increasing susceptibility to heart disease, cancer, and neurological diseases like Alzheimer's and Parkinson's.

The third main dysfunction seen with aging is a decline in the level of autophagy, a process that is regularly and strongly activated in young, healthy people but which declines in amplitude in older people. Autophagy comes from the Greek for "self-eating", which nicely describes the process. In conditions in which food is unavailable, for example overnight while asleep, and in healthy organisms, cells produce structures that degrade and "eat" parts of themselves. The structures that are targeted for destruction preferentially include old and damaged cellular organelles and proteins, and even infectious agents inside the cell such as viruses and some forms of bacteria. Autophagy is essential for maintaining our cells in a healthy and youthful state.

Autophagy normally proceeds at a low, basal level, but as mentioned a lack of food, as well as exercise and certain dietary phytochemicals, activate the process and kick it into high gear. As we age, however, our cells become less able to respond to stimuli that result in autophagy, and the process does not proceed as normal. Instead of a strong response, there is a weak one, or none at all. In this way, our cells become literally cluttered with junk, and our skin sags, organs and immune system don't do what they should, and we become increasingly susceptible to cancer and heart disease.

Oxidative stress, inflammation, and the decline in autophagy are all intimately linked in a vast network of physiological processes and enzyme and signaling systems; they all feed back and reinforce each other. How all that works is beyond the scope of this book, as it would require a vast detour into the realms of biochemistry and physiology. But suffice it to say that attacking one of these problems means attacking all of them. In this book, we will look at a number of ways to do so.

Of all of these aging processes, the decline in autophagy is perhaps the most fundamental, the most salient cause and consequence of aging. The reason for this statement is that *laboratory animals that have been subject to various genetic and chemical interventions that increase the level of autophagy live much longer than normal animals*. While they do eventually die of some other cause of aging, this shows that the decline in autophagy is probably the most important cause of aging and death. With increased levels of autophagy, decreased levels of oxidative stress and inflammation follow.

Fortunately, a number of ways exist to increase autophagy and decrease oxidative stress and inflammation, and it is possible for just about anyone to access them. The methods of attacking the problems of aging can be readily understood and are relatively easy to do. They are neither stem cell injections nor hormones. The methods that we can use to retard the aging process, and in many cases to actually turn the clock back to a more youthful state of body and mind, consist mainly of the application of various kinds of hormetic stresses. A few of them, such as the dietary phytochemicals in supplement form that we will discuss, cost something, but not much. But mostly they cost nothing other than the will and discipline needed to put them into practice.

Chapter 2: Exercise: Why It's Crucial in Fighting Aging

Regular exercise is perhaps the most powerful health-enhancing tool in the kit. If exercise were prescribed as medicine, which it hardly ever is, mortality from the top diseases would fall dramatically and billions of dollars in healthcare costs would be saved.[1] Exercise prevents older people from becoming frail and from consignment to the nursing home; it decreases rates of heart disease, diabetes, and cancer; it prevents dementia. *Anyone planning to live a long time must add exercise to his or her regimen in order to have a healthy old age.*

Exercise extends lifespan, but here we must invoke the distinction between median and maximal lifespan; exercise increases median lifespan, that is, it will help you live a full, healthy life free of illness, and as such it increases the number of people who reach the median, or average, lifespan. To attain a longer lifespan than the median, that is, to attain your maximum lifespan, you must first reach the median. It goes without saying that someone who dies of a heart attack at age 65 has attained neither his median nor maximum lifespan. Animal studies have found that exercise increases "healthspan", that is, the length of time that they live free of illness and disease, but not their maximum lifespan.[2] In humans, exercise is associated with an increase in life expectancy of up to seven years.[3] The problem here is with the word "association", since this type of study was not an experimental but an epidemiological one. Other factors, such as genes, IQ, social status, or general health can play a role in determining how much a person wants to exercise, and these factors appear to have an independent effect on lifespan. A review of studies on the effect of exercise on lifespan concluded that it does extend lifespan, but none of the studies reviewed included confounding factors (genes, etc.). The review found that endurance athletes lived longer than non-athletes, but of course excellent health may be one reason that people become athletes in the first place.[4] We'll leave all of that to one side, however, since you cannot change your genes, nor your IQ or social status (much). Most people who exercise recognize that it improves health and quality of life generally, and doctors and scientists agree.

One of the functions of exercise is to improve muscle function and strength, and muscular strength has been found to be associated with a much lower rate of cancer, with those in the top third of muscular strength having about a 40% lower risk.[5] Muscular strength is so important to cancer risk that, according to the study, the "associations of BMI, percent body fat, or waist circumference with cancer mortality did not persist after further adjusting for muscular strength." Increasing and maintaining muscle strength and muscle mass profoundly increases the odds of living in a youthful state and disease-free for a long time.

Exercise also prevents coronary heart disease, with those who vigorously exercise in their leisure time having, other things being equal, less than half the risk of heart disease compared to those who did not exercise. Those who are in the highest level of fitness, in the top fifth, have only about 20% of the risk of heart disease as the least fit.[6]

How does exercise work its magic?

Exercise is a form of hormesis which places a stress on the body and its cells; the cells then activate stress defense mechanisms so that it can withstand future stress. What happens is this: exercise increases the levels of reactive oxygen species (ROS) which act as signals to the cells. Levels of the internal antioxidant glutathione and of the enzymes catalase and superoxide dismutase increase as a consequence of the increase in ROS, as these molecules are largely responsible for protecting the body against oxidative stress, which, as we noted previously, rises dramatically with age.

In untrained people, exercise produces damage via free radicals; this accounts for the soreness and fatigue that beginners experience when they start an exercise program. But as the person continues the exercise program, the biochemical machinery that protects against oxidative stress becomes activated, and this is largely responsible for the training effect, through which the exercising person becomes adapted to his or her exercise. Regular exercise has been shown to reduce the levels of oxidized proteins and other compounds, and to increase the numbers of cellular mitochondria, both of which are very good things. (More on mitochondria below.) The paradox of hormesis explains this: causing damage (through exercise) ultimately reduces damage as the body strives to defend itself.

Antioxidants do not extend lifespan, and may even shorten it

Antioxidants, which have been touted for several decades as promoting health, actually diminish or abolish altogether the effects of exercise. In a widely cited recent scientific paper [7], scientists under the direction of Dr. Michael Ristow discovered that humans who took vitamins C and E during a program of exercise did not develop many of the beneficial adaptations to exercise, and this result has been replicated in other studies. The importance of this study lies in the fact that antioxidants such as vitamins C and E function as extinguishers of free radicals; hence, if free radicals from exercise are blunted or abolished, then no beneficial adaptations take place. In other words, the slight damage that exercise causes is intrinsic to its anti-aging effect; abolish the damage (through antioxidants) and you abolish the effect. You can't have hormesis without damage.

While vitamin C remains an important nutrient that's vital for health, taking it or other antioxidant vitamins or supplements does not prolong life, and it may abrogate the healthful effects of exercise, and by doing so potentially even shorten lifespan. Keep in mind that one sees references in popular articles and even the scientific press to "antioxidants", such as those in fruits and vegetables, when in reality they are not antioxidants, but toxic agents.

Fruits and vegetables promote health not because they contain antioxidants, but because the various phytochemicals in them produce a hormetic response, with our cells increasing stress defense mechanisms. Plants do not want to be eaten, and since they are literally rooted to the ground, they defend themselves in the only way possible, through chemical warfare. They produce chemical toxins to defend themselves from pests, including humans, and when we eat plants we ingest these toxins, which promote our health when eaten in small amounts.

Another very healthful aspect of exercise, one that retards aging, is that it increases the numbers and quality of mitochondria, the cellular organelles which are often called the powerhouses of the cell. Every cell in the body contains hundreds or thousands of mitochondria, which are the source of most of the cell's energy generation, the location in which chemicals derived from food are "burned" metabolically and used for the cell's energy needs. From this standpoint, it can be easily seen why exercise has the effect that it does on mitochondria: free radicals, increased by exercise, signal the cells to make more and better mitochondria, since more energy is required. The feeling of greater energy that a fit person or a young person has when compared to an unfit or an elderly person may largely be due to increased numbers, density, and quality of mitochondria.

Fewer and poorer quality mitochondria characterize aging cells. So characteristic is this of aging that an entire theory, the mitochondrial theory of aging, has been developed to explain the infirmities of age. In essence, as humans age, we become less able to recycle and renew our mitochondria, something that younger humans can readily do. Older mitochondria swell in size and become dysfunctional, unable to produce as much energy due to their inefficiency. In turn, inefficient mitochondria produce higher levels of free radicals and, with the internal antioxidant system also compromised by age, the cell becomes damaged. The mitochondria also damage themselves, and so, in a vicious cycle, old and inefficient mitochondria cause oxidative stress, which leads to more damaged mitochondria, more oxidative stress, and so on.

Having appropriate numbers of high-quality mitochondria is essential to attaining and maintaining a youthful physiological state.

Exercise has the capability, through the production and renewal of mitochondria, to make our bodies literally more youthful. We'll have more to say later about other tactics that can be used to keep our mitochondria in their youthful state.

Recall that autophagy is the process of self-, or cell-cleaning. Autophagy turns out to be a critically important effect of exercise, and seems to be important to its metabolic benefits such as better blood sugar control and lower insulin levels.[8] Since autophagy declines with age and is a critical factor in aging, inducing it through exercise turns out to be a brilliant anti-aging tactic. The increase in autophagy that exercise causes also connects to the renewal of mitochondria, since when autophagy increases, some of the first things the cells rid themselves of is old, degenerated mitochondria.

One of the more important sites of increased exercise-induced autophagy is the brain.[9] This has implications for brain health, as aging is characterized by declining cognitive function and dementia, including Alzheimer's disease, so increased activation of autophagy will help prevent these. We already know that physically active people are much less likely to experience cognitive decline or dementia, and a normal (high) level of autophagy is one of the main reasons for that. In essence, maintaining a high level of autophagy keeps the brain's mitochondria in a fresh and youthful state, the old mitochondria being broken down and recycled and new ones made to put in their place.

Slowing or reversing brain aging is in all respects similar to slowing or reversing aging in the rest of the body: one must maintain normal levels of autophagy, keep inflammation and oxidative stress low, and properly renew mitochondria.

Exercise also increases brain volume and the genesis of new neurons. Even an exercise as low intensity as walking can do this, increasing the volume of brain regions with both white and gray matter.[9] The brain's cognitive capacity is also increased by exercise, and increased cognitive ability means lower risk of dementia. Exercising lab animals have greater memory and learning ability, and so do exercising humans. Keeping one's mental faculties, or rather, losing them, is one of the chief worries of all of us as we get older; *exercise provides a robust defense against shrinking brain volume and cognitive decline.*

Neurons, of which the brain and nervous system is composed, secrete a protein called brain-derived neurotrophic factor (BDNF), higher levels of which are associated with both neurogenesis, or the growth of new nervous tissue, and protection against depression. Exercise increases levels of BDNF robustly, and more exercise training causes the BDNF response to increase even more than in untrained people.[10] Activating autophagy and increasing levels of BDNF appear to be the chief way in which exercise protects and improves the brain.

Sarcopenia

Another very important aspect through which exercise counteracts the aging process is through the building of muscle. Sarcopenia, which simply means muscle wasting, or loss of muscle mass and other lean tissue, is an all too common condition in the elderly, and even the not so elderly. It is a serious problem both for the individuals who have it, as well as for public health, since sarcopenia often leads to frailty, which in turn leads to falls, breaking bones, and a one-way trip to a nursing home. Healthy aging and extending lifespan entails avoiding sarcopenia at all costs.

But what causes sarcopenia? The body normally breaks down and builds up muscle continually, and the strong diurnal rhythm of autophagy is intimately involved here. When people and other animals get old, two things happen: autophagy levels decline, interfering with the proper breakdown of older cellular structures, and anabolic resistance occurs. Normally, in healthy young people, a given dose of either exercise or dietary protein has a stimulatory effect on muscle. For example, when a healthy person eats protein as part of his or her breakfast, that protein stimulates the muscle to rebuild itself from the breakdown it experienced through the previous night. Anabolic resistance refers to the phenomenon in which older people do not exhibit as intense a response in terms of muscle building to either exercise or dietary protein as do younger people. When that occurs for an extended period of time, muscles atrophy, ultimately resulting in sarcopenia.

Sarcopenia appears in aging because of increased inflammation and oxidative stress, which cause anabolic resistance. It can be quite effectively combated by two means: exercise, and proper nutrition, including enough protein. (We'll discuss protein as it relates to muscle and aging more in a later chapter.) The exercise that best ameliorates sarcopenia is the one known to academics as resistance training, and to the rest of us as weightlifting. By placing a stress on muscles, weightlifting causes them to grow, and is a sovereign cure for anabolic resistance.

Don't think that because you're not elderly, sarcopenia or muscle wasting of any kind is of no concern to you. The loss of muscle starts early in life, by some accounts before age 50, such that by age 80 most people will have lost a full 50% of their muscle mass.[11] The time to start doing something about muscle loss is when you are young.

But then again it's never too late either. Elderly people respond robustly to weightlifting, often showing dramatic increases in strength with just a few months of training. Even small increases in strength can be enough to erase frailty and keep an elderly person out of the nursing home, so this is very important.

Exercise decreases inflammation, one of the trio of major age-related physiological defects. It also increases immune response.[12] By increasing the immune response, older people can turn back their immunological clocks to that of a younger person and resist infections much more effectively. This may also have major implications for resisting cancer as well, since the immune system monitors the body's other cells for cancer and fights it when detected. One reason for higher cancer rates in the aged is due to a decreased immune response, so increasing the response can help prevent cancer.

Older men who exercise regularly do not demonstrate age-related vascular oxidative stress.[13] This type of oxidative stress is implicated in coronary artery disease, and increases with age. Regular exercise abolishes it, causing increased levels of anti-stress enzymes, and making the physiological processes in the older men's arteries like those of younger men. In this respect, that of the arteries, regular exercise stops aging in its tracks.

In summary, exercise is one of the most powerful anti-aging and longevity-promoting processes known, and anyone who wants to combat the aging of his or her body must exercise regularly, preferably daily.

The type and dose of exercise

Next comes the question, what dose and type of exercise are required to fight aging? First of all, any exercise is better than none. Being sedentary brings with it a train of illnesses and much higher risks of diseases and higher rates of all-cause mortality, or death, to us lay people. Even mere standing improves health over being completely sedentary. It's been said that sitting is the new smoking.

After standing instead of sitting, walking would be the next step up. What we want to know, however, is whether certain forms of exercise might be better at promoting longevity and retarding aging than others. The exercise that is most efficient at doing so should have certain characteristics: it should be intense enough that it causes the production of new mitochondria; it should promote maintenance or growth of muscle and combat sarcopenia; it should up-regulate levels of antioxidant enzymes. The benefits of a low-intensity exercise like walking include things like improving insulin resistance and glucose control, lowering blood pressure, and improving sleep, and those who are normally sedentary and somewhat out of shape can certainly benefit from a walking program of 30 minutes or more daily. Indeed, for the elderly or people with illnesses, this may amount to a substantial amount of exercise and be completely appropriate.

However, to get more of the benefits of exercise, it must exceed a certain threshold, which will differ depending on the person.

 To use a simple example, someone who has been training for marathons by running ten miles a day will get zero exercise benefit from a leisurely 30-minute walk. The walk that he or she undertakes simply does not rise above the threshold of intensity and energy expenditure needed to activate mitochondrial production and all of the other physiological effects of exercise, above the level that this highly trained person already has. In fact, as far as strictly aerobic exercise goes, there's likely little our marathon runner can do to make himself in better shape, since he's reached the point of diminishing returns with regard to exercise: the more exercise he does, the less effect it has.

But it's also possible to exercise too much.

Most of us do not train for marathons, and in fact, decent evidence supports the notion that a level of exercise that high is not just superfluous, but definitely unhealthy.[13] In a study of long-term runners, "strenuous joggers" had nearly double the risk of death as did light or moderate joggers. Other studies have shown that long-distance running causes heart damage[14]; fully 50% of veteran endurance athletes in one study had myocardial fibrosis, as compared to no fibrosis at all in age-matched controls[15]. The prevalence of fibrosis in these runners was not associated with their age or weight, but "was significantly associated with the number of years spent training, number of competitive marathons, and ultraendurance (>50 miles) marathons completed." Many other studies showing heart and other damage in long-term runners could be cited, but I think that the point is clear enough: it's possible to overdo exercise and take it into the realm in which it harms health. We saw in the chapter on hormesis that the health benefits of hormetic processes or substances depend on the dose, and too much of anything that causes hormesis moves the needle into the frankly toxic end of the gauge. Too much exercise damages health and will not promote healthy aging or extend lifespan. On the contrary, you may end up with a serious illness because of it.

Exercise that is too frequent can result in a syndrome known as overtraining. This is perhaps less serious than the myocardial damage that marathon running can cause, for the reason that it is usually possible to overcome it with rest and proper nutrition. Elite athletes, for instance those at the national or Olympic levels, often train so hard and so often that they become increasingly susceptible to infections, especially of the upper respiratory tract, and feel so run down and fatigued that they cannot train at the level that they and their coaches feel is optimal.[16] The cure for overtraining is backing off the level of exercise and ensuring proper nutrition, especially with regard to protein, as well as more rest. Some people report having been in a state of overtraining for years, since the idea that more and more exercise conduces to health is a popular one that mainstream health sources encourage. While, as noted, the overtraining syndrome is not as serious as the outright damage that distance running can do, if you have this syndrome you will not feel well and have more colds and flu than others; overtraining signifies too much stress and does not lead to healthy aging.

So we have an idea of the amount of exercise that goes beyond health-promoting and into the toxic range: long bouts of distance running may do this. It's unfortunate that among fitness-minded people and in the health media generally, ever longer and more strenuous running is promoted as being the way to health. It is not.

Based on the above considerations, it's clear that exercise must be intense enough to cause beneficial physiological adaptations, but not so intense, too long in duration, or too frequent to cause damage or overtraining.

Two forms of exercise seem to fit the bill when it comes to getting into that sweet spot where beneficial anti-aging actions take place, yet no damage or overtraining is done, and they are resistance training (weightlifting) and high-intensity training, often known by its acronym HIT.

Weightlifting

Weightlifting's great advantage comes from the fact that it works the entire body, and as such, it counteracts and even abolishes muscle-wasting and frank sarcopenia. Exercises like running do not involve the entire musculature, so while they do improve cardiovascular fitness, they do nothing to stop the diminishing of muscle as we age. If done properly, weightlifting also has a profound beneficial effect on cardiovascular health.

Weightlifting is not just for the bros in the gym; it can and should be done by almost everyone. To give an example of how and why this is true, consider one study in which elderly patients who had experienced a hip fracture were enrolled in a program of "high-intensity progressive resistance training", the "progressive" referring to the fact that weights lifted are increased as training proceeds. The patients also received nutritional support. Now, if elderly hip fracture patients don't meet the definition of frail, I don't know who does; a hip fracture is often a one-way ticket to the nursing home, and death within a year or so is often the tragic, ultimate result. In these patients who lifted weights, mortality was reduced by a whopping 81%[17] and nursing home admissions were reduced by 84%. Besides the tremendous magnitude of these results in terms of reducing the death rate of hip fracture patients, they emphasize the power of exercise and particularly weightlifting. Most hip fracture or nursing home residents are likely completely sedentary, which accounts for high rates of frailty and death in those conditions. Exercise turns back the clock, rejuvenating the body.

Many other studies of a similar nature have shown that virtually all elderly people can benefit from weightlifting, even into their 90s. As for younger people, a weightlifting program can prevent many of the infirmities of age from ever occurring.

Lifting weights also results in lower levels of myostatin, a protein which decreases the growth of muscle and which, in mice, is negatively correlated with lifespan. That is, less myostatin, longer life. It follows from this that the myostatin-lowering effect of lifting weights prolongs life. Other forms of exercise don't lower myostatin as much as lifting weights. How do we know this? Because less myostatin means bigger muscles, and weightlifting, along with some forms of high-intensity training, are the only forms of exercise that result in larger muscles.

While this book is not meant to serve as a weight-training or exercise manual, a few pointers about a proper weightlifting program are in order here. For the best health effects, as opposed to bodybuilding effects, weight training should focus on so-called compound exercises, which are those that involve the use of two or more joints. For example, a bench or chest press involves the use of the shoulder and elbow joints. An example of a non-compound exercise is biceps curls, in which the weight moves only around the elbows.

"The Big Five" refers to the main set of compound exercises, and these are all that are necessary for a health-promoting weightlifting program. The exercises consist of the following: 1) pull down, which works the muscles of the arms, shoulders, and back; 2) overhead press, which works the shoulders; 3) bench or chest press, which works the chest muscles; 4) rows, that is pulling weight towards oneself, which works the arm and back muscles; and 5) squats or leg press, which work the leg muscles. There's no need to get fancy with other, more elaborate exercises – although you certainly can if you want to – as these will provide all the exercise necessary for good muscle strength, better metabolism, and body weight control. If you are a beginner, some instruction is advised, as it is possible to hurt oneself if not properly trained. Older people especially should have some supervision when attempting these.

All of these exercises can be done on machines, which lessen the chance of injury, an important consideration for everyone but especially for beginners and older people. More advanced practitioners of weightlifting usually use free weights such as barbells and dumbbells to perform many of these (as I do), but that isn't necessary to obtain beneficial effects on health.

It is worth emphasizing that performing the main five compound weightlifting exercises also results in a tremendous cardiovascular and metabolic workout. Unfortunately, popular notions of exercise (which are also encouraged by health journalism) hold that weightlifting is for building muscles, but good cardiovascular and metabolic health necessitates aerobic exercise. This is just not the case. A properly structured weight workout, performed with sufficient intensity, increases cardiovascular fitness as well as does aerobic exercise, and increases metabolic fitness, as indicated by insulin sensitivity and weight loss, even better than aerobics. A recent study found that long-term weightlifters kept off belly fat much better than did long-term aerobics exercisers, so weightlifting is better for fat loss too.

How often should one lift weights? If done properly, weightlifting places a large stress on the skeletal muscles, which causes them to grow; but this large stress also means that the practitioner of weightlifting needs plenty of rest between exercise sessions. Some experts actually recommend only one session per week of weightlifting, and for older people this can be appropriate, if the exercise is done with sufficient intensity. (Walking or other less intense exercise can be used to fill in on the days in which weightlifting is not performed.) Younger people will probably find that they can lift weights several times a week without overtraining.

High-Intensity Training

High-intensity training (HIT) refers to a program of exercise that has received increasing attention from exercise scientists over the past decade. HIT takes varied forms, but in essence it involves just a few minutes of exercise a few times a week. One of the advantages of HIT is that it completely negates the excuse that most people use for why they don't exercise: lack of time. HIT has been shown to produce the same or better beneficial effects on health as other, longer forms such as aerobics or "cardio". And while most forms of steady-state exercise do little for weight loss, HIT appears to be much more effective in shedding fat.[18]

The original forms of HIT were so intense that only young volunteers could be induced to do it. But it was later discovered that the exercise need not be quite so intense to produce highly beneficial effects.[19] In six training sessions over a two-week period, markers of mitochondrial activation increased more than 50%, and markers of improved glucose control also increased. All this came about in only two weeks with a total of less than two hours of actual exercise. Other studies have shown improved glucose control in diabetics, and better insulin sensitivity in healthy young people.

HIT much more closely resembles forms of exercise that would have been done by our distant ancestors, and this being the case, we are likely to be more adapted in evolutionary terms to it. That is, our genes were meant to function in an environment in which high intensity forms of exercise were regularly done. While our forerunners undoubtedly did plenty of walking, long-distance running was probably not a regular occurrence. Instead, the demands of hunting or avoiding predators, human or otherwise, likely meant that sprinting, jumping, and lifting and carrying heavy things formed the major part of their exercise. They didn't call it exercise of course; to them it was "living".

Recall that fighting aging requires maintaining a high level of insulin sensitivity. High-intensity exercise performs way better in this category than continuous, that is, aerobic, exercise. This occurs after a single session of HIT exercise that consisted of four 30-second, all-out sprints.[20] This alone is reason enough to ditch the aerobics and do HIT.

How does one implement a HIT program anyway? In reality, the variations of HIT are limited only by your imagination. Calisthenics, for example – pushups, air squats or what we used to call knee bends, jumping jacks, burpees – can be readily combined into a HIT routine. For example, pushups for 30 seconds at as high a speed as one can do, followed by up to one minute of rest, then squats for 30 seconds, and so on. Jumping rope for 30 second intervals interspersed with short rest periods is another way. Sprinting makes for an excellent HIT routine: sprint as fast as you can for 20 to 30 seconds, walk slowly for one minute (you may need more rest time, especially at first), then sprint again, and repeat half a dozen times. These exercises are truly intense, yet take only minutes.

In the Tabata form of HIT training, the exerciser performs an exercise as fast as possible for 20 seconds, then rests only 10 seconds, and starts in again, for a total of 20 repetitions. For example, as above, pushups for 20 seconds, 10 seconds rest, then jumping jacks, and so on.

But the exact intervals and exercises do not matter as much as doing them with intensity for up to 10 minutes or so including rest intervals, and a few times a week.

A day or two of weightlifting a week with a day of two of HIT makes the ultimate exercise program: these will activate all the physiological responses necessary for peak health and long life, while avoiding the excesses of overtraining and possible damage. Naturally, those who love exercise (as I do) or who want to maximize their anti-aging will probably want to do a bit more, while also avoiding the dangers of long-distance running.

Chapter 3: Diet, or what you eat affects how fast you age

Aside from exercise, there are few more powerful agents affecting the aging process than what we eat, how much of it, and when we do so. In fact, these factors are probably *more* powerful than exercise, which is shown by the fact that exercise, or at least the type of exercise most people perform, has little effect on weight loss. (For much more on this, see my book, *Top Ten Reasons We're Fat*, 2015.) Close attention must be paid to diet in all of its permutations, that is, amount, quality, and timing, to effectively fight the aging process.

Low-fat eating is a big mistake

Let's get one thing out of the way first: the low-fat craze that the government and mainstream health authorities foisted on the American public, and which unfortunately is still followed with great enthusiasm by most health-conscious people, was a huge mistake. The rise of the obesity epidemic coincided with the adoption of low-fat guidelines, a fact that many people, and even the government, are now beginning to appreciate. The main reason for this is that eating a low-fat diet necessarily means the ingestion of higher amounts of carbohydrates, which can cause many people to become overweight or obese. Since it is becoming clearer by the day that saturated fat is not only not harmful but necessary for good health, and that the ingestion of a high-carbohydrate diet leads to overweight and diabetes, we have good reasons to believe that the low-fat diet is not optimal for human health and will do nothing to retard aging.

On the contrary, optimal anti-aging requires staying lean and along with this, sensitive to the effects of the hormone insulin. Recall that diabetes and obesity are archetypes of aging. The more body fat a person has, the higher the risk of death.[1] In general, the risks of obesity to health have been greatly underestimated, as shown by looking at mortality compared to highest ever body mass index (BMI). Popular understanding, evidenced by many mainstream articles, is that obesity isn't really all that unhealthy, but this is based on research that used BMI at time of death. However, when people die of an illness, they have often lost a great deal of weight by the time they die. When the all-time high BMI of a person is used, the mortality risk of obesity is shown to be much higher, and estimates of BMI at the time of death have substantially underestimated risks.[2]

Excess body weight accelerates aging

A recent review article by the noted anti-aging scientist Luigi Fontana and obesity expert Frank Hu took a look at all the factors relating to body mass index (BMI), and concluded that the optimal BMI was 20 to 21.[2] It's worthwhile to quote from their report: "Excess body weight and adiposity cause insulin resistance, inflammation, and numerous other alterations in metabolic and hormonal factors that promote atherosclerosis, tumorigenesis, neurodegeneration, and aging." As we've noted previously, insulin resistance and inflammation – and "numerous other...metabolic and hormonal factors" - are characteristics of aging and must be kept in check to retard the aging process. *Excess body weight accelerates aging.* Staying lean is crucial for life extension. This point cannot be emphasized enough.

Fontana and Hu go on to say, "Studies in both animals and humans have demonstrated a beneficial role of dietary restriction and leanness in promoting health and longevity. Epidemiological studies have found strong direct associations between increasing body mass index (BMI) and risks of developing type 2 diabetes, cardiovascular disease, and several types of cancer, beginning from BMI of 20–21."

In layman's terms, any BMI above 20 or 21 associates with an increased risk of the major diseases of aging. Any indications that higher levels of BMI and even obesity are healthy, as you might read in the mainstream press, are false and have come about because of faulty interpretations of the data, especially data confounded by smoking, which results in a lower BMI. As the authors state, "...maintaining a healthy weight through diet and physical activity should remain the cornerstone in the prevention of chronic diseases and the promotion of healthy aging."

Therefore, *the first objective in staving off aging is to attain and maintain a normal body weight.* All other anti-aging interventions won't make much of a difference if you are overweight or obese. Leaner is almost always better, other things being equal, than heavier. An important caveat here is that the reason that BMI means faster aging is because of excess fat, "adiposity", and not more muscle. Adding more muscle and hence attaining a higher BMI through a weightlifting program causes an increase in health, not a decrease; only more fat tissue causes a decrease in health. Health researchers can usually ignore the effect of extra muscle when doing population-based studies, since so few people have any.

A calorie is not a calorie, especially when it comes to aging

The composition of the diet matters a great deal for both lean body weight and the metabolic aspects of health. Despite what the media tells us, a calorie from one type of macronutrient (carbohydrate, fat, and protein) is not the same as a calorie from another; the body handles them differently, and levels of hormones such as insulin and glucagon, blood sugar, and muscle and fat mass are all affected by the macronutrient composition of our food. Dietary composition is of course the subject of libraries of books, so we'll narrow our focus here to aging.

To understand why the composition of our diet matters for aging, let's take a quick detour into the arena of longevity experiments in lower animals. One of the primary animals that scientists use in such experiments is the tiny worm called *C. elegans*, which has a short natural lifespan of about two weeks, allowing for faster and cheaper testing of possible anti-aging processes and substances. Many of the discoveries of the aging process in *C. elegans* were made by using genetic mutants in which specific physiological pathways were abolished.

C. elegans genetic mutants with disrupted insulin signaling can live twice as long as normal.[3] This is significant for aging in humans and for the composition of our diets because insulin is maximally stimulated by dietary carbohydrates. When we eat carbohydrates, they are broken down into glucose and enter the blood stream, and this glucose needs somewhere to go, since high blood sugar is toxic. To remove glucose from the bloodstream, the pancreas secretes insulin, which promotes the uptake of glucose into cells. *Therefore every time we eat carbohydrates, insulin signaling increases, and insulin promotes aging.*

Reduced insulin signaling also works in mice to extend lifespan; this is the means by which certain hormones, such as *klotho*, extend lifespan. Many proven anti-aging substances, such as rapamycin, both increase insulin sensitivity, meaning less insulin is produced, and increase lifespan, also in mice.

Keeping insulin signaling low is a very important component of retarding aging.

The reader may be asking whether a result like this found in worms and mice could really apply to humans. Cynthia Kenyon, the scientist who found the link between insulin and lifespan in worms, certainly thinks so; she switched to a low-carbohydrate diet shortly after she made the discovery.[4] She avoids all sugar and bread and other highly refined carbohydrates, saying that increased insulin signaling is the reason she does so. According to her, "Sugar is the new tobacco."

Other studies in *C. elegans* have found that giving them sugar *shortens* their lifespan[5] and that restricting glucose increases their lifespan,[6] so not only genetic disruption but diet directly affects aging. All of this confirms that activating insulin signaling via the ingestion of glucose has a profound effect on aging in this model organism. The physiological pathways, such as insulin signaling, are evolutionarily conserved, meaning that they are similar in the cells of all organisms. This is because these mechanisms arose early in the course of evolution, and were conserved by all subsequent evolution. For example, in mice, which are mammals like humans are, disruption of insulin signaling also increases lifespan.[7] The hormone *klotho* has been associated with longevity not just in mice but in humans, and this hormone disrupts insulin signaling.[8]

Americans eat loads of carbohydrates, by some accounts greater than 50% of their calories as carbohydrate. In fact, the Institute of Medicine, one of the arms of establishment medical consensus in the U.S., actually recommends that people eat from 45 to 65% of their calories as carbohydrate. Carbohydrates, which are composed of glucose (sugar) molecules linked in long chains, becomes sugar in the bloodstream when digested, and all that sugar has to go somewhere. To allow it to be taken up by cells, the pancreas secretes insulin which, as we've seen, is implicated in aging. When the cells receive their glucose load, they turn it into fat.

If you follow mainstream advice on carbohydrates, such as that of the Institute of Medicine, you will likely have difficulty staying lean, keeping insulin levels low, and fighting the aging process.

A common objection to the idea that carbohydrates accelerate aging is that many traditional societies eat large fractions of their diet as carbohydrates. For instance, the Kitavans, residents of a remote South Pacific island, eat up to 70% carbohydrate, and are known for excellent health; the older generations of the Okinawans are famous for long lives, and they appear to eat lots of carbs. The most likely explanation for certain anomalies like these is that these peoples ingest their carbohydrates in the form of relatively unrefined plants, which do not raise insulin levels as high. In contrast, in Western societies and other societies that have adopted Western diets, most carbohydrates take the form of flour, sugar, and processed food, much of it junk, made from these. Indeed, Kitavans, despite ingesting a high proportion of their diets as carbohydrate, have lower insulin levels than Westerners, and this may be due to the specific type of food they eat.[9] (A higher level of physical activity may also be important here.)

The lesson from the Kitavans is that any carbohydrates in your diet should come from whole, unrefined plant sources, and not highly processed forms such as flour and sugar.

Low-carbohydrate diets can lower biomarkers of aging

Low-carbohydrate diets work to lower the biomarkers of aging in humans as well as lab animals. Two of the leading physician advocates of low-carbohydrate diets, Ron Rosedale and Eric Westman, put their patients on strict carbohydrate restriction and measured some of the important biomarkers of aging, before and after. After only two to three months, insulin levels dropped by nearly half, and glucose and leptin levels dropped substantially. Their blood pressure decreased too.[10]

What does a low-carbohydrate diet look like? In the Rosedale and Westman study, the dieters were instructed that only "non-starchy, fibrous vegetables were acceptable: lettuce, greens, broccoli, cauliflower, cucumbers, mushrooms, onions, peppers, sprouts, asparagus, and seaweed." So in terms of carbohydrate, that means no bread, pasta, tortillas, rice, cereal, potatoes, or anything else that contains large amounts of starch. And of course, no added sugar. Although the dieters were not instructed to cut calories or even watch them, since this study was designed only to look at aging biomarkers and not for weight loss, they did indeed all lose weight, and average of 7 kilograms (over 15 pounds) or about 8% of their body weight. Often, low-carbohydrate diets result in a spontaneous decrease in calorie consumption, that is, these diets usually induce lower calorie intake without the dieters even trying. Usually this is attributed to better satiety: the dieters are less hungry on fewer calories when those calories come from fat and protein than when they come from carbohydrates. Sometimes, however, reports indicate that people on low-carbohydrate diets lose weight even when they do not decrease calorie intake, and if so, this is likely due to the effects of lower amounts of insulin, which decrease the storage of calories as fat and allow fat already in storage to be released from fat cells and burned for energy.

Low-carbohydrate diets can also decrease the incidence of cancer and benefit those who already have cancer.[11] Metabolic syndrome and diabetes, both disorders of carbohydrate metabolism, are associated with a higher incidence of cancer. The higher insulin levels in these conditions conduces to cancer formation; and when cancer already exists, the tumor cells feed nearly exclusively on glucose, so the higher blood glucose levels of metabolic syndrome and diabetes encourage their survival and growth. Ketone bodies that result from very low carbohydrate diets can negatively affect the proliferation of tumor cells. Since cancer rates increase dramatically with age, cancer being essentially a disease of older people, the fact that low-carbohydrate diets can decrease cancer rates is yet another indication of their pro-longevity and anti-aging effect.

How low is a low-carbohydrate diet? Definitions are disputed, and the issue is important because of studies that have reported no difference in weight loss or aging biomarkers such as insulin on low-carbohydrate as compared to low-fat diets. It appears that some researchers are happy to deem a diet with 40% or greater calories as carbohydrate as a low-carbohydrate diet, merely because that's lower than the average consumption, or because of researcher bias, or even because they mistakenly believe that going lower than that is unsafe. So a categorization here is important.

A group of prominent medical scientists in the area of obesity and diabetes have suggested the following definitions for low-carbohydrate diets[12]:

- Ketogenic low-carb: This is the lowest of the low-carb, and results after a few days in the production of ketones, which many parts of the body use for energy in place of glucose. On a ketogenic diet, carbohydrate consumption is less than 30 to 50 grams per day.
- Low-carbohydrate diet (full stop): Anything up to 130 grams of carbohydrate per day.
- Moderate carbohydrate diet: more than 130 grams but less than 45% carbohydrate as calories, which on a 2,000 calorie a day diet equates to about 225 grams.

Any decrease at all in carbohydrate consumption will have beneficial effects on aging biomarkers, but greater restriction is usually better, and many people do very well on a ketogenic diet. Anything above 130 grams of carbohydrate a day, a "moderate carbohydrate" diet, is not really restricting carbs in the way we mean here.

Later in this book, we'll be discussing the benefits of fasting, but it's worth noting here that many of those benefits are due to the restriction of dietary carbohydrate.[13] A group of volunteers underwent a fast of 84 hours – that's three and a half days, a very long one. Half of them received intravenous infusions of a lipid emulsion that met their daily energy requirements. Yet ultimately, changes in glucose, insulin, free fatty acids, and other biomarkers were the same in both groups, the study's authors concluding that "restriction of dietary carbohydrate, not the general absence of energy intake itself, is responsible for initiating the metabolic response to short-term fasting." Not all relevant biomarkers were measured, but this makes the case that the mere lowering of carbohydrate intake has many health benefits.

The science behind insulin signaling and lifespan is complex, and by no means have the discoveries come to an end or all the difficulties been ironed out. But what I have hoped that this brief tour through insulin signaling and lifespan shows is how an anti-aging diet must be a low-carbohydrate diet. In humans, low-carbohydrate diets result in lower insulin levels and better insulin sensitivity. All carbohydrates eventually become glucose in the bloodstream, and this causes the release of insulin. While it is absolutely required for life, too much insulin shortens life. Other manipulations such as exercise and fasting that fight aging also increase insulin sensitivity.

Dietary Phytochemicals

While dietary carbohydrates are a net negative for decreasing disease and increasing lifespan, a number of dietary constituents play a positive role in lifespan extension, many of these constituents being polyphenols and other compounds derived from plants, which are generally known as phytochemicals. A fairly large number of compounds extend life in *C. elegans*, and others also in mammals such as mice, and since so many exist, we'll focus here on those that show the biggest benefit or the most promise. Note also that most foods contain relatively low amounts of many of phytochemicals, and so if you want to use them for life extension purposes, supplements are often the best way to get them.

Many or most of these plant phytochemicals work by increasing the activation of AMPK, which is a highly evolutionarily conserved cellular energy sensor. AMPK senses the energy status of cells, becoming more activated when energy levels are low, and when activated it in turn regulates gene expression, increasing stress defense mechanisms and making for efficient metabolic control. Ultimately, it controls the aging process through its integrated cell-signaling network.[14] Therefore, activation of AMPK slows, stops, or even reverses aging, and if we can activate it using phytochemicals (or other agents, of which we'll discuss more later), then we can slow or stop our own aging.

In the past few decades, a huge amount of research has been devoted to a great number of plant compounds that have beneficial health effects, such as the prevention of the diseases of civilization like heart disease and cancer. Over 10,000 potentially beneficial phytochemicals exist, many of them having not been characterized well. Many fruits and vegetables are loaded with them, but as noted they may be difficult to obtain in sufficient concentration in the diet, and most studies have been done using relatively large doses of these compounds, large enough that humans would need supplements of them to obtain a sufficient amount.

Probably more research has been done on resveratrol than any other phytochemical that promises to halt aging. Resveratrol is found in red wine, although the amounts there are small, about 5 milligrams in a bottle. It extends lifespan in a number of model organisms, including the nematode (worm) *C. elegans*, and promotes survival in mice fed a high-fat diet.[15] Resveratrol promotes the production of mitochondria, improves insulin sensitivity, prevents cancer, and enhances the beneficial effects of exercise, and one of the main reasons, if not the only reason, for its beneficial health effects is through the activation of AMPK.

Most of the work on resveratrol has been done on lab animals, but some human trials exist, and have had good results[11], with this compound functioning as a calorie restriction mimetic. As we'll see later, calorie restriction is one of the most powerful anti-aging strategies, and ways exist, such as the use of resveratrol, to mimic its actions. These mimetics dispense with all that pesky hunger that characterizes calorie restriction.

While resveratrol isn't quite the cure-all for aging that many had hoped in the beginning, it's well worth supplementing with. In the cited human study, the scientists used a dose of 150 mg a day, and they stated that, "although the dosage of 150 mg of resveratrol per day is around 133- to 266-fold lower compared to the high doses of 200–400 mg/kg/day used to supplement mice, plasma resveratrol levels in our human intervention...were even higher than those obtained in mice". This is important to note because of reports that the human body metabolizes resveratrol too quickly for this compound to be effective. This human study showed that it is not. Resveratrol lowered systolic blood pressure by about 5 mm, a substantial amount, it increased mitochondrial activity, and of course increased activity of AMPK. While the results were not miraculous, they show that resveratrol has essentially the same action in humans as in animals.

Resveratrol causes increases in memory and cognitive function in humans.[17] As a decline in brain volume occurs during aging, maximizing brain power and preventing brain shrinkage becomes an important part of fighting aging. One doesn't want to live to an old age if it means substantial brain shrinkage – at least, I don't. Resveratrol activates the anti-aging gene klotho[18] and has substantial anticancer effects.[19] The doses used in most human studies have approximated 150 milligrams daily; this dose appears safe for humans and is the amount this writer takes daily.

Other chemical compounds can also activate AMPK and thus mimic calorie restriction, for example, curcumin, which is derived from the Indian spice turmeric. Curcumin extends lifespan in C. elegans, fruit flies, and in mice, and it appears to do so in part by promoting autophagy, the cellular process of self-cleaning. It inhibits inflammation, and prevents cancer by activating stress defense mechanisms, i.e. through hormesis. Sulforaphane is another such compound with similar activities; broccoli and other cruciferous vegetables contain relatively large amounts of it.

One problem in aging that scientists would like to solve is that of cellular senescence. As cells age, they enter a stage known as senescence, in which they cease to grow and divide like normal cells. Their senescent phenotype does, however, produce large numbers of inflammatory cytokines which can cause many of the hallmarks of aging. The problem of senescence differs from some of the other biological problems of aging discussed in this book in that it is not readily overcome through the easily available anti-aging agents of diet and exercise. Now, though, it looks like a dietary phytochemical has come to the rescue, in the form of quercetin, which is found in sources like apples and onions.[20] In a recent study, quercetin showed remarkable effects on cellular senescence, and improved the health of old mice after a single dose.[21] While quercetin was effective, the best results were obtained in combination with an anti-cancer drug, dasatinib. While the researchers cautioned that this is all very preliminary, and that much more research is needed, the results show the promise of using dietary phytochemicals like quercetin to fight aging.

Eating a diet high in fruits and vegetables allows for the consumption of a wide range of beneficial dietary phytochemicals, and with them the possibility of preventing cancer, heart disease, dementia, and other diseases of aging. Other dietary components also contain high levels of beneficial phytochemicals, notably coffee, tea, chocolate, and red wine, all of which have been shown to improve health. Caffeine has in fact been shown to extend lifespan in *C. elegans*. Supplementation can increase the level of selected phytochemicals, and from the above list, this writer supplements both resveratrol and curcumin, which provide for hormesis.

Coffee is the single largest source of phytochemicals for the average American, who doesn't appear to be eating many of his or her fruits and vegetables. The upside of that is that coffee does provide high levels of polyphenols, and recently it was found that coffee induces autophagy[22]; therefore coffee promotes longevity. Coffee drinking is also associated with greatly decreased risks of diabetes.

Consumption of tea, especially but not exclusively green tea, has also been associated with longer life, and much of its life-extension and health-promoting power likely comes from its phytochemicals, mainly catechins, such as the nearly unpronounceable epigallocatechin gallate, which fortunately we can refer to by its initials, ECGC. This phytochemical promotes autophagy, and has increased lifespan in mice.[23] In rats, EGCG caused a 13% increase in lifespan, and the longer-lived animals had decreased levels of oxidative stress and inflammation.[24] The dose of EGCG used in these rats was 25 mg per kilogram of body weight, which translates into a human dose of about 220 mg a day, assuming a 70 kg (154 lbs.) person, and taking the rats' higher metabolism and surface to volume ratio into account. This dose is easily achievable with a green tea supplement of 400 mg, which contains ECGC of about 200 mg.

Other chemical compounds exist which extend lifespan in lab animals, but which are almost impossible to obtain with food, lithium, for example. Lithium not only increases lifespan in C. elegans, but humans who drink high-lithium water have lower death rates.[25] Lithium is also a somewhat mysterious required nutrient, and it appears that the recommended daily allowance is about 1 mg. (Which is, by the way, far lower than the dose used in bipolar disorder, which is hundreds or even thousands of milligrams daily.) If you don't have lithium in your water, and most people don't, a supplement is needed here; lithium orotate, a common formulation, is available in 5 mg tablets, and could be taken, say, every other day or every third day.

The daily use of low-dose aspirin, that is, the size of a baby aspirin or about 80 mg, is associated with a reduction in risk of certain cancers, notably colon cancer, in humans of about 40%. Reductions in risk of esophageal cancer were a whopping 75%. (Higher doses of aspirin show no additional benefit, but may have higher risk.) Aspirin also extends lifespan in *C. elegans*[26] via activation of AMPK. Aspirin has of course been used for years in the prevention of heart attacks, but it carries with it the risk of major bleeding, so doctors have been generally reluctant to recommend it to anyone who is not at high risk for heart disease. However, that may be changing, since adding the lowering of cancer risk to the equation means that the risk to benefit ratio of aspirin has changed. Peter Rothwell, the medical scientist and physician who has done many of the studies on aspirin and cancer risk, now takes aspirin himself, despite having no known cardiovascular risk factors, and has said, "In terms of prevention, anyone with a family history would be sensible to take aspirin". (From the *New York Times*.) Some anti-aging experts believe that aspirin could be the easiest and cheapest life extension drug now available, since it has a demonstrable effect in lowering mortality.

Aspirin has two different effects.

The first is that it lowers the risk of cardiovascular events like heart attack and stroke by reducing the chance of blood clots, which are the precipitating factors for these cardiovascular diseases. It does this by reducing the ability of blood platelets to stick together and to other surfaces. This effect is also the same one that may cause bleeding.

Aspirin's second effect is that it lowers inflammation by inhibiting certain enzymes and activating the energy sensor AMPK; this is the source of its anti-cancer and anti-aging effects. Recall that one of the hallmarks of aging is greater levels of inflammation, so a drug like aspirin that reduces inflammation can be of benefit for life extension. The tendency of aspirin to promote internal bleeding is certainly a downside, and some people will be more likely than others to manifest this risk. But the reduction in cancer risk may be even more important than the reduction in cardiovascular risk. The medical consensus currently recommends aspirin only for those who have had a previous heart attack or are otherwise at high risk for one, but as noted that consensus may be changing. For those of us who are trying to fight aging, aspirin poses a conundrum: any doctor that you might consult about taking low-dose aspirin will likely recommend against it, assuming that you have low cardiovascular risk. I'm not here to tell you otherwise, but you should be aware of aspirin and what it can do.

Omega-3 fatty acids, which are abundant in fish oil, are another dietary component important to aging. Modern, industrial diets are loaded with omega-6 fats, mostly from vegetable oils, and this has skewed the ratio of omega-6 to omega-3 fats far in excess of what our distant ancestors experienced. Excess omega-6 fats are associated with cancer and heart disease. Aside from limiting the intake of vegetable oils, preferably to zero, supplementing with fish oil can help bring the balance of omega-6 to omega-3 back to normal. A teaspoon of cod liver oil is about 5 grams and contains about one gram of omega-3 fatty acids. Taking this amount a few times a week should be sufficient for anti-aging purposes.

Omega-3 fatty acids lower levels of inflammatory cytokines, thus lowering one of the three main biomarkers of aging. They also have salutary effects on the brain, and may also aid in exercise recovery.

Dietary Protein

We mentioned dietary carbohydrate above, and noted that, for anti-aging purposes, generally speaking the lower the amount of carbohydrate in the diet the better. Lowering the level of carbohydrates in the diet improves insulin sensitivity, which notably declines with age, and improves weight control. There is no dietary requirement for carbohydrates, so they may be decreased or omitted from the diet with no ill effects and in fact for most people, great benefit.

Protein is another matter: it is a required nutrient and we cannot live without it. Low protein levels may lead to all kinds of functional difficulties and illness, from frailty and sarcopenia to chronic fatigue and depression. Vegetarianism is, for example, associated with a number of health problems due to its low protein content, and many vegetarians report a distinct lack of energy, and is one reason some of them give up on their vegetarian diet.

The Growth-Longevity Trade-Off

However, in the context of life extension and fighting aging, it is possible to eat too much protein. The reason is that a fundamental trade-off between growth, on the one hand, and longevity, on the other, exists. More growth equals more aging, other things being equal. Protein raises the levels of insulin-like growth factor, or IGF-1, which is, as the name suggests, a type of growth hormone. IGF-1 acts in a number of ways and is connected to many other cellular and biochemical sensors, but in essence it promotes growth. In doing this, the body's natural anti-aging programs, such as the AMPK sensor, which affects autophagy, inflammation, and oxidative stress, are shut off. Higher levels of IGF-1 are associated with cancer and earlier death, and centenarians appear to have lower levels of growth hormones.

People who have genetic mutations that cause growth hormone receptor deficiency essentially have very low levels of growth hormone, insulin, and IGF-1 effects on their cells, and they appear to be nearly free of diabetes and cancer.[27] They have "a major reduction in pro-aging signaling", and serum from these people even reduced DNA breaks and increased apoptosis (killing of cancerous and pre-cancerous cells) in cell culture. Growth hormone receptor deficiency also leads to much higher levels of insulin sensitivity, which decreases with aging and leads to diabetes and other diseases of aging.

Unfortunately, growth hormone deficiency also causes very short stature. Unless you are one of the few who is indeed very short, we don't need to worry about this though, as we're already fully grown. The key is to maintain growth hormone signaling at a lower level once adulthood has been reached.

Growth signaling fundamentally links to pro-aging biochemical pathways. Block or diminish the growth pathways, and pro-aging signaling decreases, and with it the risks of the diseases of aging: heart disease, cancer, diabetes, and the rest.

Why does the trade-off between growth and longevity exist? Lots of speculation has gone into this question; one answer is that genes which are necessary for growth, such as IGF-1, are not turned off sufficiently in later life, and thus cause cellular senescence and other pro-aging phenomena. IGF-1 is absolutely necessary for normal growth and development: mice lacking it die after birth, and as noted those people with growth hormone receptor deficiency are very short in stature.

The existence of hormones and other substances and processes that promote growth while an organism is maturing, and which promote aging when an organism is older, has led some scientists to propose the idea that aging is *quasi-programmed*. The organism has a necessary physiological program that causes growth and is unable to completely shut it off later. Whether this theory is true or not, it does seem to fit the facts of the growth-longevity tradeoff.

Many anti-aging clinics and doctors advocate the supplementation of human growth hormone (HGH) as an anti-aging intervention. (As well they might, since it's expensive and they can make lots of money from it.) Provision of HGH superficially decreases markers of aging by lowering levels of body fat and increasing muscle mass, and many of those who take HGH report higher levels of energy and well-being. However, this comes with a price, as higher HGH actually accelerates aging by, for example, increasing insulin resistance; by causing growth, HGH can also increase the rate of cancer and probably heart disease as well.

The effects of HGH seem paradoxical, for how can a hormone both increase markers of aging, such as insulin resistance, and decrease other markers, such as those involving body fat and muscle, at the same time? Science doesn't have all the answers to this yet, but the tradeoff between growth and longevity appears inescapable.

As we'll discuss in much more detail later, calorie restriction is one of the most robust anti-aging interventions in existence; it's been known since the 1930s or even earlier that feeding animals drastically less food, say 30% less, increases their lifespans dramatically, sometimes by up to 50%. Much research and speculation has gone into understanding why this occurs, but one way calorie restriction works is through lowering levels of growth hormone and IGF-1. The way that calorie restriction appears to lower the levels of these hormones is through lower protein intake. Many of the benefits on lifespan of calorie restriction disappear if protein intake is not lowered, and even the deficiency of a single amino acid (of which proteins are composed), methionine, increases lifespan in rodents, even without calorie restriction.[28]

The effects of calorie restriction and protein intake in humans on IGF-1 was nicely illustrated in a recent study. Researchers measured levels of IGF-1 in a group of people who belong to the Calorie Restriction Society and who had been restricting their food intake for a number of years. Since calorie restriction must be accompanied by good nutrition in order to be effective for anti-aging purposes, these people had been very conscientious about their protein intake, and consumed a diet that was around 24% protein, or 1.67 grams of protein per kilogram of body weight. This level of protein intake is high, similar to that consumed by bodybuilders. (By contrast, most people consume around 15% of calories as protein.) Their IGF-1 levels averaged 194 nanograms per milliliter (ng/ml), a level similar to that in people eating a standard, non-calorie restricted diet. Then, they cut back on their protein consumption to around 1 gram per kilogram for three weeks, and their IGF-1 levels dropped to 152 ng/ml, a drop of about 25%.[29]

The precise levels at which IGF-1 either lowers or promotes aging in humans is not known, so we can't say with certainty that either the higher level that came with higher protein promotes aging, nor that the lower level fights it. However, all things considered lower levels are probably better. The important point about this study is that at least in humans, calorie restriction by itself does not lower IGF-1 levels, and protein is a key determinant of those levels. The authors of this study remark that "reduced protein intake may become an important component of anticancer and anti-aging dietary interventions."

To be fully aboard the anti-aging program, attention must be paid to how dietary protein and other habits and interventions affect the levels of growth hormone and IGF-1.

Protein and muscle

We need to consider another aspect of protein intake and how it relates to aging, and that is the issue of muscle-wasting and sarcopenia. We saw earlier that muscle wasting begins early in life, and that the continuation of this wasting into old age can result in sarcopenia, or the loss of enough muscle mass to make people frail and their lives difficult. Protein, along with exercise, also determines the level of muscle mass, so people need to eat enough protein to maintain muscle and avoid frailty in older age.

Optimal protein intake involves balancing the two desirable factors of 1) avoidance of muscle wasting (and even increasing muscle mass); and 2) keeping IGF-1 levels from being too high. This is especially important if you do resistance training, since that won't increase muscle mass without sufficient protein.

Fortunately for the goal of increasing lifespan, the amount of protein needed to build muscle appears to have been exaggerated. Most weightlifters use an approximation of 2 g protein per kilogram of body weight – compare to the admittedly low U.S. recommended daily allowance of 0.8 g/kg – but this appears to be much more than necessary. A number of studies have found that experienced weightlifters need only about 1 g/kg.[30. This study is representative of others that found similar results.] Trained athletes need less protein than beginners, as the body adapts to use protein more efficiently with training. Also, keep in mind that these were experienced bodybuilders who were maintaining a large muscle mass; for those of us not quite so zealous in muscle building and maintenance, less protein than that may suffice. In this particular study, the authors concluded that "bodybuilders during habitual training require a daily protein intake only slightly greater than that for sedentary individuals in the maintenance of lean body mass".

Interestingly, endurance athletes such as runners require much more protein than strength athletes, probably because this type of exercise tends to break down muscle through higher levels of cortisol, among other things. All the more reason to make resistance training the core of your exercise regimen.

Muscle growth appears to be much more linked to lower levels of myostatin, a protein produced during exercise, than it does to increased systemic levels of IGF-1. A quote from a study called "Resistance training alters plasma myostatin but not IGF-1 in healthy men" gets to the heart of this matter: "... growth factor responses local to the muscle may be more important than circulating factors in contributing to muscle hypertrophy with resistance training."[31] Large systemic increases in IGF-1 are unnecessary to promote hypertrophy of our muscles; decreasing myostatin levels does the job. Therefore, at least as far as IGF-1 goes, we don't need as much protein.

The lesson in all this is to keep protein intake under control, neither too much nor too little. *Insufficient protein conduces to sarcopenia, and with it to frailty and dependence; too much protein leads to higher levels of IGF-1 and faster aging.* Based on what has been set out above, we can tentatively state that a daily protein intake of a bit above 1 gram protein per kilogram of body weight may be about right. This amounts to around 0.5 grams per pound of body weight. Anything more than that, other than for beginning weightlifters, is likely superfluous and leads to faster aging. Lower than that, it may lead to muscle wasting. This level is still above the recommended daily allowance for protein, which is 0.8 grams of protein per kilogram of body weight, and which has been criticized as being too low.[32]

How can we optimize the amount of protein we eat? Aside from counting the number of grams, an easier way may be to eat enough protein on exercise days, and to lower protein consumption on non-exercise days. (By non-exercise days, I don't mean days that incorporate low-intensity exercise like walking, which requires no extra protein, but weightlifting or HIT days, which do.) Fasting, wholly or partially, on non-exercise days can accomplish this, and we'll explore this in more detail in the next chapter.

Chapter 4: Fasting: When you eat is as important as what you eat

Diet, in the sense of the composition and quality of the food we eat, is rightly emphasized as important for health and lifespan. Low-carbohydrate diets impede aging by curtailing insulin resistance and obesity, and added sugar can degrade health and accelerate aging. The amount of protein, as we have seen, can make the difference between muscle-wasting and frailty, on the one hand, and faster aging on the other. And of course optimal health and lifespan extension require adequate supplies of vitamins and minerals. Health experts routinely blame the obesity epidemic on changes to our diets, especially the consumption of more refined carbohydrates including sugar, and in this they are surely correct, at least in part.

Most people used to fast regularly, because they had to

Besides the quality and composition of our diet, another aspect of food may be equally or even more important for our health, levels of body fat, and aging, and that is the matter of when and how often we eat.

Looking at the obesity epidemic, is it the case that most people followed impeccable eating habits before the epidemic began? And is it also the case that scientific knowledge of what humans should eat and how that affects health was greater than today? Certainly, the answer to both of these questions is "no". Before the 1970s, when the obesity epidemic began, most people not only didn't have a clue as to how food affected their health, but they didn't care all that much either. Before the 1970s, cakes, pies, and cookies featured regularly in Americans diets; sugary cereal was (and still is) eaten regularly for breakfast, and soda pop from a vending machine was never far away. So how did most of the population avoid being overweight or obese, unlike today?

The answers to that question are complex, and most of them lie outside the scope of this book, but one aspect of eating that has changed is the timing and frequency of meals. Think back to the *real* old days, long before the 1970s, when refrigeration didn't exist. In those days, food was difficult to store, and leftovers didn't last long. No convenience foods either. The wife and mother of the household prepared meals for her family from scratch, and this was a time-consuming job. Restaurants were fewer and most people couldn't afford them anyway.

What changed? We now not only have refrigeration, but frozen and packaged convenience foods aplenty. Fast food restaurants are everywhere, and many more people can afford them and have access to them. Eating a meal or snack now is as close as the refrigerator or cupboard – no wives or mothers necessary – or a drive a few blocks to the nearest McDonalds or other fast food joint, where the food is cheap. We are now able to eat around the clock, and we do so.

Surely the increased availability of food bears some responsibility for the obesity epidemic.

Before the current day, people regularly fasted, going without food for perhaps 12 hours between dinner and breakfast. Snacks were not as readily available, so most people ate only at meals.

Fasting, or going without food for some arbitrary amount of time, not only helps keep us lean, but as we're about to see, also has a powerful influence on health and lifespan, and is possibly the most potent instrument currently available for this purpose. It's free and has no toxic side effects, and can be done by almost anyone.

To understand how fasting can extend healthy lifespan, we'll start with the science behind calorie restriction, the most robust intervention for fighting aging known to date. These effects have been known, if not understood, for hundreds of years and possibly longer.

Calorie restriction extends lifespan

In the introduction to this book, I mentioned a man who discovered calorie restriction in the 16th century and successfully applied it to his own life, managing to live past the age of 100 in an era when hardly anyone at all did this. That man was Alvise, or Luigi, Cornaro (1467-1566 – sources vary on his age at death, with some sources reporting 102. In any case, whether 99 or 102, he was very old.)

Cornaro was an Italian nobleman who became wealthy enough to have Tintoretto paint his portrait. At the age of 35, he found himself with "a heavy train of infirmities"[1] that he believed were caused by "too freely eating and drinking, to which I had been addicted", and which included a "disordered" stomach, "and I suffered much pain from colic and gout, attended by that which was still worse, an almost continual slow fever, a stomach generally out of order, and a perpetual thirst. From these disorders, the best delivery I had to hope was death." It sounds very much like he had a case of diabetes, which in the case of type 2 diabetes can indeed be caused by excessive eating and drinking. Excessive fructose intake causes gout, from which Cornaro suffered, and this is a feature of the consumption of sugar, which is half fructose.

If Cornaro was not near death, he certainly felt like it and almost wished for it, so much was he suffering from ill health. His physicians had little to help him, until one suggested that he eat and drink sparingly. Cornaro, "feeling it was my duty as a man to do so", immediately undertook to eat only 12 ounces of food daily, "neither more nor less", and to drink 14 ounces of wine, or a little over half a modern bottle. His meals, other than wine, consisted of meat, poultry, eggs, fish, bread, and vegetables. His infirmities quickly disappeared, and he resolved to live that way the rest of his life, which he did. Worthy of note also is Cornaro's declaration about how his "sober life" improved his disposition, that he was "freed by God's grace from the perturbations of the mind", and that he no longer experienced any "contrary emotions".

The physician who suggested to Cornaro that he eat sparingly may have been the recipient of a long line of knowledge that went back an undetermined number of years or centuries; but we can never know that for sure. (Fasting as a cure for illnesses dates back to Hippocrates.) But Cornaro may be the first case of a man cured of his illness and allowed to live a long life through restriction of food, or at least he's the first one we know about.

The modern study of calorie restriction began with a project of the scientist McKay in 1930, who discovered that rats fed less food lived substantially longer than rats fed "ad lib", that is, who ate all they wanted and at any time.

Calorie restriction, or CR as we'll refer to it, works on many fronts to prolong healthy lifespan, and scientists are still unraveling the biochemical and physiological mechanisms by which it does so. In essence, CR acts as a stress on the organism, that is, it's a form of hormesis, and the body reacts by up-regulating stress defense mechanisms.

CR involves the feeding of 30 to 50% fewer calories to lab animals than they would normally eat, or want to eat. When started early, CR can extend lifespan up to 50% in rodents, and decreases levels of oxidative stress, inflammation, and mitochondrial dysfunction, and helps maintain youthful levels of autophagy. It also lowers levels of insulin and the growth hormone IGF-1, which is important to its mechanism of action.

In what physiologists refer to as the "fed state", which is just what it sounds like, the period of time when food is being digested and its components being shuttled to the various places that need it, insulin and IGF-1 levels are increased, and this abolishes the cellular self-cleaning process of autophagy. In the fasted state, with no food being taken, autophagy is strongly up-regulated, allowing cells to rid themselves of accumulated junk. CR is actually a form of partial starvation, and this has the effect of increasing autophagy. Since one of the functions of autophagy is to provide nutrients for the organism when none other are available, it's not difficult to see why CR increases it.

Calorie restriction means cleaner, younger cells

As mentioned, decreased stimulation of insulin and IGF-1 is believed partly responsible for the mechanism of action of CR. It turns out that animals with selective mutations, or knockouts, in genes for insulin and IGF-1 signaling live much longer than normal animals. The physiological mechanism here is that lower levels of insulin and IGF-1 cause decreased stimulation of the mammalian target of rapamycin (mTOR), which in turn means increased levels of autophagy.

Higher levels of autophagy mean that animals, and the cells of which they are composed, continually rid themselves of accumulated junk, such as malfunctioning mitochondria, glycated proteins, and other cellular components that have passed their expiration date. They then replace these structures with newly manufactured ones, and in this way, autophagy results in younger cells, and a younger organism. Maintaining autophagy levels in their youthful state is critical for lifespan extension, and based on the state of scientific knowledge at present, the most important physiological process in retarding aging and stopping the clock.

Many scientists have expressed great enthusiasm for CR with regard to lifespan extension, and with good reason.

However, CR is not without its drawbacks.

For one thing, many people will find the prospect of reducing their calorie intake by 30% or more to be daunting, if not repugnant. Those reading a book on anti-aging are in a minority, and while they may be willing to consider CR, most people will not. (This writer is one of those uninterested in practicing CR.)

The other drawback of CR is that if it isn't done with precision, ensuring complete nutrition with minimal calories, and sometimes apparently even if it is, then malnutrition, frailty, and immune deficiency can be the result. For example, it's recently been found that CR in mice has "distinct but deleterious consequences to the aging immune system"; in particular, mice subject to CR were much more prone to infection than normally fed mice.[2] Since a declining immune system is already a feature (or a bug) of older age, and since infectious diseases take quite a toll on older humans, if these results translate to humans (and there's no reason why they would not), CR may not be a very good strategy for lifespan extension. This comes with the caveat that particular forms or modalities of CR may be discovered that do not have a deleterious effect on the immune system. That remains to be seen.

There's also concern that CR could lead to brittle bones, a low muscle mass, and other consequences to physiological systems that are already at risk in older people.

Intermittent fasting, the CR alternative

An alternative to CR exists, one that has virtually all of its benefits and perhaps even more, and that has practically no downside, and that is intermittent fasting. The practitioner of intermittent fasting merely goes without food for some prescribed amount of time, which can vary greatly. Fasting has the great advantage over CR that lower calorie intake doesn't necessarily feature in it. Animals and humans typically eat the same amount of food, or perhaps just slightly less, as do ad lib fed animals and non-fasting people. They do this because during the so-called feeding window, that is, the time during which food may be taken, they make up for lost calories during fasting by eating more. Almost the only difference is in the timing of eating. Therefore, *intermittent fasting does not have the downsides of reduced immune function or malnutrition and frailty*.

In fact, one can even build muscle on a regime of regular intermittent fasting, and many bodybuilders have taken to fasting, as evidenced by the popular bodybuilding website Leangains. It's even better for fat loss, another aspect of body composition to which bodybuilders pay close attention.

Fasting may effective for both improved health and longer lifespan because our evolutionary history has caused humans to be adapted to it. Many animals that are high on the food chain might eat only once every few days, after a kill. Human hunter-gatherers certainly do not eat breakfast, lunch, and dinner, interspersed with snacks; rather, the typical pattern seems to be the hunting and gathering of food during the day followed by a large meal at night when the food has been prepared. If our genes are indeed adapted to bouts of fasting, then our usual pattern of three meals a day plus snacks could interfere with our physiological makeup and lead to the diseases of civilization.

The practice of "grazing", that is, eating every two or three hours, long said to be healthful and useful for keeping off excess body fat, is in reality a harmful practice that you should stop, whether or not you plan to fast. The impetus behind grazing seems to be the idea that it will maintain blood sugar and metabolism at a higher level; *in reality, grazing just makes people fat*. Along with the low-fat dieting craze, grazing must be one of the more harmful of recently invented dieting practices. Grazing promotes aging.

Mark Mattson, a leading scientist in the study of aging, along with colleagues, studied mice subjected to alternate-day fasting.[3] In this form of fasting, the animals were fed no food at all on one day, and allowed to eat as much as they wanted the next, and this schedule was repeated continually. They found that their food intake did not decrease and they maintained the same body weight as mice fed ad lib. The authors stated that "intermittent fasting resulted in beneficial effects that met or exceeded those of caloric restriction including *reduced serum glucose and insulin levels and increased resistance of neurons in the brain to excitotoxic stress.*" (My emphasis.) These results show that intermittent fasting has beneficial effects on metabolism and on neuronal stress resistance that is independent of the amount of food intake. So judging by this study, restriction of food intake isn't necessary to retard aging, so long as the timing is right.

Intermittent fasting also causes increased heart rate variability in rodents, as well as increased resistance to myocardial infarction (heart attack) and stroke.[4] Heart rate variability has come to be seen as a key sign of the integrity and youthfulness of an organism; when the heart responds to minor stimuli with a minute variation in rate according to the organism's needs, this is a sign that all physiological systems are finely tuned and in optimal condition.[5] Intermittent fasting causes increased resistance to heart attack and stroke by up-regulating the transcription of genes that encode for cellular antioxidant and other stress defense mechanisms. As before, there's no reason why all of this should not apply in humans as well as rodents.

Intermittent fasting also exerts profoundly beneficial effects on the brain and nervous system, and it has been suggested that this regimen may be very useful in the prevention and treatment of Alzheimer's and Parkinson's diseases, two of the specters of old age. [6] One of the ways in which it does is through increasing the levels of an important protein, brain-derived neurotrophic factor, or BDNF, which allows the brain to maintain its plasticity and ability to grow new neurons and make new neuronal connections. In senescence-accelerated mice, intermittent fasting allows them to maintain normal levels of BDNF, in contrast to their well-fed counterparts.[7]

In a study of experimental congestive heart failure in mice, intermittent fasting led to vastly increased survival compared to their ad lib fed counterparts, at 88.5% vs 23%, a 3.5 fold difference. [8] It would be no exaggeration to say that this magnitude difference in survival is amazing.

We see that intermittent fasting can prevent insulin resistance, improve brain function, and even increase survival from congestive heart failure, and is a profoundly anti-aging regimen. Increased insulin sensitivity, which results in increased levels of autophagy, is key to the benefits of fasting.

Short-term fasting results in profound neuronal autophagy in mice. [9] The scientists who discovered that fasting causes autophagy in the brain and nervous system state, "Our data lead us to speculate that sporadic fasting might represent a simple, safe and inexpensive means to promote this potentially-therapeutic neuronal response." Fasting rids the brain of junk and allows it to be healthier at an older age, essentially rejuvenating it. For many of us, keeping our brains in a youthful state will be reason enough to practice intermittent fasting.

Intermittent fasting: schedules and durations

The duration of an intermittent fast can vary greatly. Unfortunately, human data on the effects of various lengths of time of fasting regimens is lacking, but we can make some educated guesses. For starters, we know that in healthy young people, an overnight fast of perhaps twelve hours is enough to strongly initiate autophagy. We also know that a decline in levels of autophagy is prominent in aging and perhaps the most important correlate of it. Therefore, older people, that is, anyone beyond say the decade of his or her twenties, should consider fasts of longer than twelve hours if they want to maximally activate autophagy and turn back the aging process.

A very common method and duration of intermittent fasting as it's currently practiced is sixteen hours in length, with the only missed meal being breakfast. In this version, one eats a regular dinner at the regular time, at perhaps 6:00 P.M. Then, nothing else is eaten until about noon the next day, resulting in a sixteen to eighteen hour fast. This fast is easily done, and this writer does it regularly. Coffee or tea are acceptable to drink during a fast; purists might take them black, but small amounts of cream – but not half-and-half, as it contains milk – are acceptable, as cream, which is 100% fat in calories, only very weakly activates insulin signaling and thus will not interfere with the health benefits of your fast. Coffee itself activates autophagy, so this may be a bonus, and both coffee and tea are well-known for appetite suppression, so either or both of these may make a fast easier. This writer considers coffee and tea essential for fasting.

Should one wish to, this fast can be extended into the afternoon or evening, for a 20 to 24 hour fast, and others extend their fasts even longer, up to 36 hours. Beyond this length of time, it is no longer really an intermittent fast, but a prolonged one, which we'll discuss in a moment.

Intermittent fasting of sixteen to twenty hours can be done daily. Another way of looking at it is the inverse, that is, the length of the feeding window, that time during which you allow yourself food. A daily feeding window of eight hours ought to allow for a strong increase in autophagy during the fasting phase, and results should become apparent in a few days to a few weeks. Many people of course use fasting to lose weight, and if you have this as a goal, keep in mind that the existence of a feeding window doesn't give permission to eat anything you want and still lose weight. Those for whom losing weight is not a goal need not restrict the quantity of food they eat during the feeding window, although attention to quality is highly recommended, as eating junk food and/or lots of refined carbohydrates could negate many of the beneficial effects of your fast. Many bodybuilders who use fasting for fat loss are in the habit of taking branched-chain amino acids (BCAAs) or whey protein during their fast in order to prevent any loss of muscle, and this is an acceptable practice for that goal. But BCAAs or whey will completely abolish autophagy, so if you're fasting for the health benefits, namely increased autophagy, do not do this.

If losing weight is one of your goals in undertaking intermittent fasting, many people find that it's an easier regimen than dieting. With dieting, constant attention must be paid to the type and quantity of food being eaten, and many dieters fail for the reason that this attention can be difficult to adhere to over long periods of time. With fasting, you simply don't eat, and you know what you're going to do well ahead of time: if it's a fasting day, or if it's currently during your fasting window, you don't eat. Simple.

Some of the initial difficulty in intermittent fasting is psychological. In fact, probably most of it is. So many of us are used to eating every few hours or whenever the fancy strikes us that deliberately going without food for any stretch of time seems unnatural. Most of us have never gone any length of time without eating, and have never even skipped one meal. The practice of snacking is ridiculously widespread; it's as if the body wasn't designed for going without food for even a few hours, which of course it is.

Most people seem to think that fasting is crazy. If you're going to practice intermittent fasting successfully, you will simply have to ignore what anyone else says about, and do your own thing. You will however have the satisfaction of becoming healthier and leaner than those around you.

Prolonged fasting

Beyond intermittent fasting, more prolonged fasting has also been advocated by several medical researchers, perhaps most prominently by Valter Longo, a scientist who studies aging and fasting at the University of Southern California.[10] Longo emphasizes that he prefers the health effects of fasting to calorie restriction, as he does not believe that restrictions on the amount of food over a longer term are good for most people. Much of his work has centered around the effect of fasting on retarding the growth of tumors, and he has also shown that several days of fasting can prevent the bad side effects of chemotherapy.[11] Fasting for several days strongly lowers levels of insulin and IGF-1, and this likely accounts for its benefits. Prolonged fasting also has been shown, in mice, to promote regeneration of the immune system.[12] Autophagy, as we've discussed, removes cellular waste, and in the case of prolonged fasting whole cells of the immune system are broken down. These cells are then replaced with new ones, and immunosuppression is reversed. Prolonged fasting essentially has the ability to make the entire immune system young again.

Cancer patients may be of course more highly motivated to undertake fasts of this length than the rest of us, and probably most people won't be willing to fast for a number of days strictly for life extension purposes, although I've met people who have done so. One great motivator for many people to undertake prolonged fasts is fat loss, which these fasts do quite well. The well-known health blogger and advocate for low-carbohydrate diets, Jimmy Moore, undertook a 7-day fast.[13] The data on prolonged fasting as it affects aging is sparse, but given adequate nutrition, and provided that they are not done too often, are likely very effective in combating aging, and in particular they lower IGF-1 and insulin levels a substantial amount. To get effects such as the regeneration of immune cells, longer fast such as these may be necessary.

Fasting, whether intermittent or prolonged, is generally quite a safe thing to do. There may be some people, however, who need to be careful and also may need a doctor's supervision; these would be people whose health is not generally good, such as the very overweight, or those with serious illnesses such as heart disease and cancer. Diabetics may need to alter the doses of their medications, so these folks should always consult a doctor before beginning any fasting regimen.

If you already eat a relatively low-carbohydrate diet, hunger pangs that may come with fasting are easy to overcome. It's been remarked by many people that on a low-carb diet, one does not experience hunger in the same way as when eating high-carb. That sounds strange, but it's been my experience too, and when fasting, hunger doesn't really bother me much. One comes to enjoy the sensation; in fact, the increase in various hormones and neurotransmitters during fasting may contribute to a sense of well-being and even elation.

Autophagy enhancers and inducers

The fact that fasting fights aging through boosting autophagy has led some scientists to study autophagy enhancers or inducers, chemical substances that activate autophagy, which these scientists refer to as calorie restriction mimetics, although they could just well be called fasting mimetics.[14] Among these are the over-the-counter weight loss aid hydroxycitrate, which induces "massive" autophagy in mice. Other compounds that induce autophagy are nicotinamide (a form of vitamin B3), resveratrol, curcumin, and EGCG, a compound abundant in green tea and probably responsible for most of its health benefits. The study of autophagy inducers is in its infancy, yet the compounds listed here all have a good safety profile. It's probable that small doses of these taken during a fast will enhance the already increased autophagy. This isn't a recommendation, but I'm putting this information out there because these compounds have promise in inducing and increasing autophagy, and thus may have true anti-aging effects. Some of them, namely resveratrol, curcumin, and EGCG, have been shown to extend life in lab animals, and it wouldn't surprise me if hydroxycitrate turned out the same. This writer has used 300 mg of hydroxycitrate during fasting, as well as nicotinamide at 500 mg.

Hydroxycitrate, resveratrol, and curcumin (but not nicotinamide, to my knowledge) have all been shown to have anticancer properties. In my view, this is likely intimately linked with their ability to promote autophagy.

Staying in tune with human evolutionary heritage through fasting will result in better health and will retard aging. The aforementioned

Mark Mattson has written of "challenging oneself intermittently for health".[15] Humans and those from whom they are descended evolved in environments in which there was scarcity of food, a high level of fitness was required in order to hunt and fight, and dietary phytochemicals which contain toxic elements were eaten and from which physiological defense mechanisms must defend us. As a result of not challenging ourselves, through a sedentary, couch-potato lifestyle and the constant eating of processed food high in refined carbohydrates and devoid of dietary phytochemicals, we are in the midst of an epidemic of diabetes and obesity.

The burning of fat for energy, as opposed to the use of glycogen, is one of these adaptations. Glycogen is the storage form of carbohydrate, and our bodies typically carry only about a one-day supply of it. By contrast, even lean people have enough fat on their bodies to keep them supplied with energy for weeks. (The apparent world record for fasting was made by an obese man of about 450 pounds who fasted for over a year and lost some 250 pounds in the process. He was medically supervised, it is worthwhile to note.)

When we graze, and never allow ourselves to enter the fat-burning mode, we're in a physiological state which our ancestors did not experience much of the time, and as a consequence become ill and overweight. The restoration of ancestral conditions, in part through fasting, allows gene expression to proceed in the proper way, and can restore health and prolong lifespan.

Chapter 5: Demolition and Renewal: The Optimal Anti-Aging Strategy

Our bodies are like cities

The fabric of a city is composed of buildings and other infrastructure, which organically evolve to suit the needs of its inhabitants over time. A city of today typically looks nothing at all like the same city of one hundred years before. Buildings that are no longer useful have been torn down in order to make room for new ones in their place. The buildings themselves have been constantly renovated with new roofs and furniture and plumbing. Even without advances in technology or increases in population, cities must still be renewed in this way because things simply wear out.

The city in this analogy is like the body of an organism. The body one has today is not the same body one had last year, and even more so the same one as decades ago. The cells of which the body is composed, as well as the furniture and plumbing in them, the organelles and proteins and other elements, have been replaced in a process of controlled demolition, and new ones erected in their place. Some parts of our bodies are rather static, such as the bones and the brain, but even these have a degree of plasticity that allows for renewal. Other parts, such as skeletal muscle, skin, or the cells that line the intestines, are more responsive to environmental conditions such as nutrition and exercise and can turn over in the process of self-renewal much more quickly.

But, like a decaying civilization that can't manage to maintain its cities, so that these cities accumulate rubbish, the buildings become decrepit and unusable, and the roads narrowed or blocked, aging makes bodies become less adept at tearing down older structures as well as less able to erect new ones in their place. This inability for self-renewal is perhaps the most important hallmark of aging.[1] While other markers and pathologies of aging, such as insulin resistance, oxidative stress, mitochondrial dysfunction, and systemic inflammation, are important to the aging process, they are all correlated to a decline in autophagy, the process of demolition that clears the way for renewal.

Increased levels of autophagy through calorie restriction or fasting or genetic manipulation extend the lifespan of animals more than any other intervention known. The word "intervention" is an important one here, since this means that we can modify at least this particular aspect of aging. Fixing other aspects of aging, such as increasing telomere length or renewing stem cells are more difficult and so far have only been done in laboratories, and in any case seem to be of less critical importance than kick-starting autophagy.

Increasing autophagic activity requires no expensive drugs nor consultation with a doctor in an anti-aging clinic. It does require a bit of self-discipline, and the knowledge of how it all works will help keep you on the right track. So here's a bit of that knowledge, hopefully not too full of science jargon, that will help guide the reader.

As mentioned, autophagic activity declines with age. Can we get an idea of how great the decline is? In some studies, very old rodents had about one-sixth the autophagic activity of young ones.[1] Human data on this is lacking, but it's clear enough that such a decline exists and that bringing levels of autophagy up to those of young people is necessary if not sufficient to slow aging.

Dysfunctional mitochondria have been thought to play a major role in aging, so much so that scientists came up with a mitochondrial theory of aging.[2] Mitochondria are the cellular organelles often referred to as the cells' powerhouses, since their function is to produce energy for the cell and the organism as a whole. Mitochondria that have passed their sell-by date produce a higher level of free radicals, which damage both the mitochondria themselves as well as surrounding cellular structures. In addition, they are unable to produce as much energy, which is manifested as, among other things, physical fatigue. In essence, dysfunctional mitochondria cause the cell as well as the organism to which it belongs to become old and rundown. Ultimately, whole organ failure can result.

Autophagy targets old, dysfunctional mitochondria

One of the principal tasks of autophagy is to break down old, malfunctioning mitochondria. The cell can sense which mitochondria need to be broken down, and selectively targets them. When autophagy doesn't function at a high level, as in aging, the old mitochondria remain in place, emitting free radicals and generally poisoning the cellular environment. Increasing autophagic activity, other things being equal, means that an older person will have better renewal of mitochondria and a cleaner, more youthful cellular environment.

Free radicals, or reactive oxygen species as they're technically known, were also long thought to be critical to aging through the damage they cause. The late Denham Harman developed this theory, but newer research shows that it cannot be the fundamental cause of aging, since cells require reactive oxygen species for signaling purposes, and since some animals have high longevity coinciding with high levels of oxidative damage; the naked mole rat is one such animal. Increased levels of free radicals are also part of the response in hormesis, and hormesis is a healthy, anti-aging process. (This also explains why antioxidants have such a dismal record in life extension, not only not working, but perhaps even harmful.) In light of the previous section on mitochondria, and in light of the fact that old mitochondria are the main sources of free radicals, it can also be seen that free radicals are not the fundamental source of pathology in aging, but rather a consequence of it.

Why antioxidants won't help

Oxidative stress and inflammation are also two very important pathologies in aging. As we noted above, free radicals or reactive oxygen species are required by cells for signaling, so abolishing free radicals through supplementation of antioxidants or any other method is not on the program, since cells don't even do this when the organism is in its youthful state. Instead, cells and the organism strive to maintain reactive oxygen species in balance, neither too many nor too few.

To maintain oxidative balance, an elaborate, internal antioxidant mechanism exists, of which the small peptide molecule glutathione is quantitatively and qualitatively the most important. Glutathione quenches free radicals and becomes oxidized, and is itself then recycled back into its active, reduced form. When the glutathione system is overwhelmed by too many free radicals, and when it cannot be replenished quickly enough or at all, the antioxidant system is overwhelmed, too many free radicals damage cells, and a state of oxidative stress is said to exist.

In a normally functioning, youthful organism that has access to good nutrition, excess free radicals cause an increase in antioxidant enzymes, including those that deal with the production and recycling of glutathione. Substances and processes that cause hormesis, for example exercise and dietary phytochemicals, cause an increase in free radicals and consequently an increase in glutathione and other antioxidants. Abolishing the free radical signal, for example through the provision of relatively large amounts of vitamin C, can also abolish the healthy hormetic effect of physical stressors, as seen in the suggestively titled study "Antioxidants prevent health-promoting effects of physical exercise in humans".[3] Those free radicals are an essential part of becoming healthier.

In organisms that are not functioning normally, or in aging organisms, the internal antioxidant system that produces and recycles glutathione may not react properly to increased levels of free radicals, and oxidative stress occurs. Why does this happen? One reason cells cannot respond properly is if they are unable to make enough glutathione. As this molecule is a small tripeptide, that is, it's composed of three amino acids, and amino acids in turn are derived from protein, an insufficient intake of dietary protein can ultimately lead to insufficient glutathione.

Glutathione is critical

To get to the heart of the matter of increased oxidative stress as it relates to aging, we need to dig a little deeper into glutathione, what it is, and how it's made. The three amino acids of which glutathione is composed are cysteine, glycine, and glutamine. Cysteine is the rate-limiting constituent in glutathione synthesis, meaning that the cellular machinery can only produce glutathione if sufficient cysteine is provided; the other two amino acids are usually present abundantly. As the organism ages, cysteine becomes less available for glutathione synthesis, and this is so characteristic of aging that it's been asked whether aging is a syndrome of cysteine deficiency. [4] It may very well be.

Cysteine becomes less available in aging because it is partly the job of autophagy to supply it, and autophagy declines in aging.

During periods when no food is available during fasting, even overnight fasting, the body must maintain a balance of nutrients, electrolytes, and chemical gradients that allow it to function normally. This is the process of homeostasis. When the organism goes without food long enough, autophagic activity increases, and tissue, especially skeletal muscle, is partially broken down, and the molecular components that result from the breakdown of tissue are used to supply the other cells and to maintain homeostasis. In the case of skeletal muscle, the main components supplied are amino acids, one of which is cysteine, and that cysteine is used to make glutathione. When autophagy doesn't proceed at a level appropriate for the organism, which occurs in aging, then cysteine is in short supply, and not enough glutathione is made.

Therefore a decline in autophagy can lead directly to increased oxidative stress.

Skeletal muscle is an amino acid storage organ

Skeletal muscle, in addition to its other functions, acts a kind of storage organ, whose function is to retain amino acids from protein consumption for later use, when no protein is available. It builds itself up when protein is consumed, and beaks itself down through autophagy when it is not.

A lack or decrease in autophagy means that muscle fails to perform one aspect of its storage function, since it cannot release amino acids for use.

Levels of glutathione actively fluctuate inside the body, the turnover in young healthy people being close to 100% in one day.[5] In comparison, in elderly people the turnover is about half of that, that is, the rate of synthesis is lower. Overnight, glutathione levels can drop substantially because of this. To compound a shortage of glutathione, many people, especially the elderly, do not eat enough protein and thus have even less cysteine available for glutathione synthesis.

The result of all this, a lower level of autophagic activity in the elderly leading to less cysteine and lower glutathione, is increasing oxidative stress, since not enough glutathione is available to mop up excess free radicals. It can be seen that oxidative stress in aging, which is highly characteristic of it, can ultimately be traced back to lower levels of autophagy.

Cysteine supplementation

Cysteine supplementation can partly compensate for low autophagy and relieve oxidative stress, and supplementation is relatively easy. [5] The inexpensive over-the-counter supplement n-acetylcysteine (NAC) supplies cysteine; it is rapidly absorbed from the gut, taken up by cells, where it is de-acetylated, and the resultant cysteine used for glutathione production or other uses for which it is needed. Whey protein, a supplement used enthusiastically by bodybuilders, is rich in cysteine, and provision of whey protein can increase levels of glutathione, whereas casein, the other main milk protein, does not.[6]

The cysteine content of whey is about five times higher than that of casein, the other protein component of milk, and also much higher than in meat. (In case you were wondering, whey is the protein fraction of milk that remains when milk has been curdled in preparation for making cheese. The casein protein curdles, the whey stays liquid. Until recently, with the increase in use of protein powders, cheese producers practically gave it away.) We'll discuss whey supplementation below.

Oxidative stress, which virtually everyone older than 30 has to some degree, and which radically increases in old age, can be relieved with NAC supplementation.[7] Elderly people, aged between 60 and 75, had their glutathione levels measured, along with levels of plasma hydroperoxide, which is a measure of oxidative stress. The level of oxidative stress in the elderly was about 40% higher than in younger control subjects, and levels of glutathione were about 50% lower. After supplementation with NAC for 14 days, as well as with another component of glutathione, glycine, levels of both oxidative stress and glutathione became nearly identical to levels in the young controls.

To banish oxidative stress in older age, it is critical to maintain proper intake of the amino acid cysteine, which helps to maintain glutathione.

The most important way to maintain high blood levels of cysteine, and therefore ensure high (appropriate) levels of glutathione, is through the process of autophagy. This is how nature does it, and by keeping our recommendations in tune with nature and amplifying nature's dictates, we stand the best chance of remaining in health and fighting aging. As we've copiously noted, autophagy declines with age, and is one of the chief correlates of age. The lower your level of autophagy, the older you are physiologically, regardless of your chronological age.

The main way to increase levels of autophagy is through fasting. Now, younger people with a finely tuned physiological apparatus have no trouble in this area. Overnight fasting is enough to strongly activate autophagy. Critically important is that one of the most important products of autophagy is cysteine. When skeletal muscle tissue is cleansed through autophagy, and old, dysfunctional cellular structures and proteins are targeted for recycling, amino acids appear in the bloodstream, one of which is cysteine. The other cells in the body, mainly those of the liver, take up cysteine and use it to make glutathione. So the levels of glutathione increase, and oxidative stress decreases.

As we age, we need more than just an overnight fast to activate autophagy to levels useful for life extension purposes. The same amount of time fasting that strongly induces autophagy in the cells of a young person will not do the same in an older person. But if that older person extends the amount of time fasting, then he or she can activate autophagy to levels normally seen in younger people, and this is key.

As we've seen in previous chapters, fasting activates autophagy quite strongly.

To combat aging, autophagy should be activated and/or enhanced in such a way that it amplifies its normal circadian rhythm. To do this, we will extend our overnight fast into the next day. By how much is a good question, but I suggest that we aim for a minimum of a 16-hour fast, and do this regularly, even every day if you can handle it.

Others may want to lengthen their fasts even more. Many people do 24-hour fasts, some do 36, and others even longer. (But as noted, this gets into the area of prolonged, not intermittent, fasting, which is another kettle of fish.) This writer currently fasts for 16 hours two to three times a week. I do occasional fasts of 20 to 22 hours, from 6:00 P.M. one evening, after dinner, to around 4:00 P.M. the next day, and this hasn't been terribly difficult at all. One of the secrets to eliminating hunger is to drink coffee and tea, which won't spoil your fast, and I take full advantage of this effect.

Autophagy boosters, such as hydroxycitrate or nicotinamide may be appropriate during your fast. I often take either 250 milligrams of the over-the-counter weight loss aid hydroxycitrate or 500 milligrams of nicotinamide (vitamin B3) midway through my fast in order to amplify fasting's effects on autophagy. (Interestingly, the weight loss effects of hydroxycitrate has been found to depend on its activation of autophagy, probably through activation of AMPK, the cellular energy sensor. This likely causes an increase in fat-burning. That's speculation at this point though.)

If you worry about losing muscle mass during a fast, you shouldn't. Calorie restriction in middle-aged lab animals actually means that they retain muscle and have improved muscle function.[8] Intermittent fasting is a better intervention than calorie restriction, since generally it entails the same number of calories ingested as for animals and people who eat all they want. It's even possible, using the right strategies and schedule, to increase muscle mass all the while practicing intermittent fasting. We'll discuss how to do that shortly.

Fasting causes a strong increase in levels of growth hormone, and the body does this in order to preserve muscle and bone. Meals actually suppress production of growth hormone.[9]

Diabetics, or anyone with issues of blood sugar control such as hypoglycemia, should consult a doctor before engaging in fasting. Fasting longer than overnight is also inappropriate for growing children, who need the calories and protein to ensure their proper development. For most other people, fasting for relatively short periods poses little risk, but when in doubt, consult your doctor.

The title of this chapter is "Demolition and Renewal", and since we've discussed the process of controlled demolition, which is autophagy, we'll now discuss renewal.

The renewal of the body in aging

Renewal involves building up new structures in place of the old ones. To do this, good nutrition is a must, and in particular, the right kinds and quantity of protein are necessary. For example, we've seen that cysteine is a critical component for the maintenance of our body's internal antioxidant system, because glutathione production requires it. The other essential amino acids, that is, those that the body can't make for itself and must be ingested in the diet, should also be optimized.

Protein can be characterized by biological value. Biological value refers to the proportion of essential amino acids a protein contains, and higher biological value means just what it sounds like, organisms thrive and grow better on protein of higher biological value. If a protein is of lower biological value, then the body can use only a fraction of that protein, since the proportions of amino acids don't match the body's needs.

Animal proteins are always of higher biological value than vegetable proteins. Whey protein has the highest value, at an index of 104, with milk at 91, and beef at 80.[10] By contrast, wheat gluten comes in at 64, and soybeans at 74. There's also a digestibility factor to be accounted for, the details of which we need not go into here, but when this is taken into account, vegetable sources of protein fare even worse. For instance, whey comes in at 1.00 on this scale, gluten at 0.25.

Does this mean that vegetarians have trouble getting enough, good quality protein? Not necessarily, but it may be difficult for vegans, who do not eat any animal products at all. While this is not the place to get into the entire debate surrounding omnivorous versus vegetarian diets, staving off the ravages of aging means eating at least some animal protein, in my opinion. The reason for that is the phenomenon of muscle wasting.

We've seen in previous chapters that sarcopenia, or muscle wasting, is one of the main maladies of aging, and strongly to be avoided, as it leads to frailty and nursing homes and in many cases, death. Most 80-year-olds will have lost 50% of their lean body mass – replaced in most cases with fat. Muscle wasting also occurs to some degree starting at relatively young ages unless we take measures to stop it. Eating high quality protein is one such measure.

Sarcopenia occurs gradually. A small imbalance between breaking down and building up muscle, a phenomenon which happens daily, can over a long period of time result in sarcopenia. Since one leg of our anti-aging program is to encourage the body's normal mechanisms of breakdown and amplify it, we must carefully balance that with properly building everything back up. And if we don't supply the right quantity and quality of protein, that won't happen.

Scientists have long debated, and still debate, how much protein humans need. The topic is necessarily complex, since protein requirements depend on things like the presence and amount of other macronutrients like carbohydrate and fat, the energy status of the person – for example, whether he or she is currently gaining or losing weight – and the health status of the person. Certain illnesses and injuries, such as burns and trauma, greatly increase the body's protein requirements. For the purposes of this discussion, we'll assume that the reader has no major illnesses, wants to build and retain muscle, remain in optimal health, and retard the aging process.

Now, bodybuilders definitely want to build and retain muscle, and most of them eat very high amounts of protein. They are also, other things equal, in excellent health. (That is assuming they don't take steroids or other performance-enhancing drugs.) But it's been found that even trained bodybuilders require about 1.1 grams of protein per kilogram of body weight.[11] If bodybuilders get by on that amount of protein, then the rest of us can also. Note that this amount of protein is still above the recommended daily allowance (RDA) of 0.8 gram so protein per kilogram of body weight, which has been criticized as too low. People who eat this amount of protein, 0.8 g/kg, can lose lean muscle mass, and below that level things become even worse, with lower immune function and increased oxidative stress, for example.

Shooting for a protein intake of above 1.0 grams per kilogram, and below 1.5, might be optimal. This way we're sure to be able to retain and build muscle, but without radically increasing levels of IGF-1, which promotes aging.

Most people will have little trouble eating this amount of protein, so long as one follows a paleo(ish) diet, relatively low in carbohydrates, that features some form of animal-derived protein at each meal. Meat, fish, eggs, yogurt (without sugar), all have high levels of high-quality protein. Wheat gluten, which some vegetarians promote as an alternative protein source, does not make the cut.

If you are vegetarian, I strongly recommend that you include some animal protein sources in your diet. These sources could be, for example, whey protein powder, other dairy products like yogurt, or eggs. As for veganism, I'm afraid that I don't recommend it for a number of reasons. Humans did not evolve to eat that way, and protein intake on a vegan diet will almost necessarily be inadequate. There are no vegan societies and apparently there never have been, so that should give us a strong hint about the viability and desirability of being vegan. Sorry, just the truth as I see it.

To build ourselves up, we also need exercise. As pointed out in a previous chapter, exercise is a sovereign cure for many, many ills, and someone who doesn't exercise cannot expect to live a long, healthy life. (A few people with superior genetics seem to manage; the rest of us need to work at it.) But as I also pointed out, resistance training (weightlifting) and high-intensity training (HIT) are superior forms of exercise, superior because they result in much better muscle mass and retention and better metabolic control. Aerobic exercise can help retain muscle, but not nearly so well as lifting weights and HIT.

Of course, some older people may not be able to engage in these activities as much, although resistance training has been shown to be effective in people into their 90s. Assuming that one has some degree of infirmity or frailty, walking for exercise is completely appropriate, and should be engaged in daily. Walk for at least a half hour at a decent pace, and increase this with time if possible. If one is so infirm that one can't do this, a supervised exercise program specially designed for very old or infirm people may be an alternative.

For the rest of us, not so old and not so infirm, we should lift weights and do high-intensity training.

In weightlifting, concentrate on the big compound lifts, which exercise large parts of the body and provide a good metabolic and cardiovascular workout. The big compound lifts are comprised of bench or chest press, military or shoulder press, rows, pull-downs or pull-ups, squats, and dead lifts. This isn't the place to go into all the details of a weightlifting program, but a little further detail may be helpful.

These exercises may all be done on machines, and for the beginner that's probably the best course of action, since machines minimize any chance of injury. Using free weights (barbells and dumbbells) requires a certain level of skill and coordination, which many older people may not have, and which many others might not care enough to learn. (Popular books on weightlifting seem to assume that everyone wants to learn to squat 300 pounds.) A little instruction from a decent book or from a personal trainer will be helpful. My own weight workouts are done using a combination of free weights and machines, but I'm a little more serious about my weightlifting than the average person.

If you lift weights, added exercise in the form of HIT may not be necessary. That is because weightlifting itself, if done with sufficient intensity and with short rest periods in between sets, is a form of high-intensity training itself, resulting in a great metabolic and cardiovascular workout. While I still do some form of HIT once in a while, my main exercise when away from the gym is walking. Weightlifting requires plenty of rest, and in fact one book on the topic (*Body by Science*) recommends lifting weights only once a week. I like to lift more than that, but that means one needs even more rest, so normally I don't perform exercise of high intensity on my off-gym days.

A word to the women in the audience: all of this applies to you too. If as a woman you are concerned with building too much muscle and becoming masculine looking, stop worrying. Building muscle to the degree that well-built men have requires not only tons of hard work, but lots of testosterone too. Women have only about one-tenth the level of testosterone that men do, so building large amounts of muscle is very difficult for women. As for the level of work, men who seriously try to build muscle spend many hours a week of very difficult training doing so. Building muscle isn't easy. So get into the gym – or get a set of weights to use at home – and lift. You may be surprised at how welcoming the guys in the weight room are.

High-intensity training of the sort that includes working all parts of the body also builds muscle, although not to the same degree as weightlifting does. But HIT of this type will almost certainly be enough to retain muscle and to avoid sarcopenia and frailty. So when you do HIT, make sure to include exercise like pushups, burpees, squats (knee bends, we use to call them), dips, and sprints. These, while not making you look like Arnold, will keep muscles in fine shape as well as help keep you lean with a low percentage of body fat.

Weightlifting and other intense exercise should be followed by food, and fasting should not follow exercise. This is essential to the building-up phase of our anti-aging program. Eat high-quality, unprocessed food along with high-quality protein in the 24 hours after a bout of hard exercise. (We can exclude walking or other relatively less intense exercise from this stricture.) The body can't build muscle and repair itself without food.

Whey protein is ideal for building muscle after a workout. Taken either right before or right after a workout, whey raises levels of critical, essential amino acids in the bloodstream and strongly promotes muscle synthesis. Some studies have shown that whey taken at other times of the day, hours before or after the workout, does not promote muscle building, but other studies dispute this, and the matter is still open for debate. But it seems a good precaution to drink your whey near the workout, either within one hour before or one hour after.

As for other food in the 24 hours after a workout, meat, eggs, yogurt, and the like will all help build muscle.

Ideally, one should not contemplate starting a fast until at least 24 hours after hard exercise. Resistance exercise strongly up-regulates levels of muscle protein synthesis for about 24 hours after the bout of exercise, so it's important to get proper nutrition in that time window.

Synthesis: breakdown and renewal

Putting all of this together, our optimal anti-aging strategy cycles between fasting and feeding, and the feeding period coincides with the time in which we want to exercise. Fasting means controlled demolition through autophagy, the cellular self-cleaning process, and renewal is the building of muscle and the maintenance of cardiovascular and metabolic health through exercise.

Our body normally cycles this way too, with controlled demolition occurring during the night when we do not have access to food, and rebuilding during the day, when we do. *Our strategy merely amplifies natural, physiological cycles so that they proceed like they do in young people.*

In young people, the cycles of breakdown and renewal are like sine waves, with high peaks and low valleys, and they proceed without much help or input from the person. In older people, that is, anyone older than his or her twenties, the peaks begin to decrease and the valleys begin to rise, so that the sequence of sine waves that represent breakdown and renewal are flattened. To return these sine waves of breakdown and renewal to their normal, youthful configuration requires interventions, and the most important of these will be intermittent fasting, on the one hand, and proper exercise and nutrition, on the other.

Variations in schedules of intermittent fasting and feeding/exercise can be nearly infinite, so one can only offer examples that may be useful. Here is a sample schedule, one that the author follows.

Day 1, morning: Exercise consisting of weightlifting at the gym. Either before or immediately after my workout, 25 grams of whey.

In the following 24 to 36 hours, meals with decent quantities of high-quality protein, such that I take in >1 gram of protein per kilogram of body weight.

Day 2: In the evening, following dinner, fasting begins, with nothing to eat until much later on the next day.

Day 3: Fasting. Coffee in the morning, tea at mid-morning. Depending on my daily agenda and other things, like how I'm feeling, I may fast until 4 P.M., making a total fasting duration of 22 hours. If I have things to get done, or if I'm feeling less than energetic, I may fast only until noon, making my fast from 16 to 18 hours long. Then I eat several good meals.

Day 4: Back to the gym for a workout, and then the feeding phase. Etc.

This schedule works well for me. In this way, I can properly attend to the renewal of my body's resources ion the form of building up muscle. I then have plenty of time to be properly fed to assure that the renewal proceeds optimally. Then, every third day, I maximize the activation of autophagy through fasting, assuring that the cells of my body will rid themselves of dysfunctional mitochondria and outdated proteins. I help to ensure that IGF-1 levels remain in a lower range, thus helping to prevent cancer, diabetes, heart disease, and other aging maladies.

Different schedules may work better for others. One variation sometimes practiced is a weekly fast of 24 hours or more. This variation will strongly promote autophagy, yet it will leave one free to exercise and feed on all other days and perhaps even go to a party or two, all without overthinking the schedule. A recent popular diet book promotes alternate day fasting on two days a week, and this might also be rather convenient.

Intermittent fasting is also great for fat loss, and those with some pounds to lose shouldn't hesitate to try it. However, one word of caution is to be careful during the feeding windows. If you eat as much or then some during feeding as you omitted when you fasted, or if diet quality is poor, fat loss may be slow to non-existent.

Chapter 6: Conclusion

Aging represents the decline in functional capacity of the organism and the increasing susceptibility to disease. Scientists who study aging have greatly enlarged our understanding of aging, yet we still do not know its fundamental cause. In theory, there seems to be no reason why we should age at all, or why we shouldn't live forever, barring accidents or predation. When we are young, the body repairs itself and recovers from injury easily; the decline in our ability to repair ourselves is at the heart of aging.

To combat aging and live long enough to see actuarial escape velocity, we need to recover our ability to repair ourselves. Until the day comes when technology can mend the molecular structure of the cell, our own repair mechanisms must suffice. We must keep our repair mechanisms in good repair.

To do this, we must understand the evolutionary pressures that formed the current human genome. Our genes evolved in an environment in which meals were irregular and fasting for hours to days happened regularly; in which dietary phytochemicals promoted the hormetic up-regulation of cellular stress defense mechanisms, and in which vigorous physical activity, not sedentary behavior, was the norm. To achieve health and to have a shot at retarding aging, we can't be couch potatoes living on junk food, whose only recreation is hours of watching television.

The guidelines for fighting aging in the best way we currently know are:

1. Stay active. Sedentary behavior was all but unknown to our human ancestors. If you work long hours at a desk, consider a standing desk, or at a minimum take regular breaks for brief exercise. Being active is an important part of a lifestyle in which hormesis plays a role.

2. Stay lean. Even having just a little extra fat on your body causes an increase in levels of inflammation and oxidative stress, which can also lead to insulin resistance, metabolic syndrome, and diabetes. The physiology of obesity is the archetype of pro-aging. The optimal body mass index (BMI) is around 20 to 21, somewhat higher if you lift weights and add muscle.

3. Beyond just staying active, exercise. Exercise combats inflammation, oxidative stress, and mitochondrial dysfunction, three of the hallmarks of aging, and increases autophagy to youthful levels. Consider doing the most healthful forms of exercise that have the biggest anti-aging effects, weightlifting and high-intensity training.

4. A low-carbohydrate diet is an anti-aging diet. Strive to eat <20% of daily calories as carbohydrate, and eat paleo style: no sugars, grains, legumes, or vegetable oils. Don't eat processed junk.

5. Include ample dietary phytochemicals in your diet. Main sources of these include cruciferous vegetables (such as broccoli), berries (such as blueberries), chocolate, tea, coffee, and red wine.

6. Consider supplementation with select phytochemical supplements, such as resveratrol, curcumin, and green tea extract. These promote hormesis and up-regulate cellular stress defense mechanisms.

7. Dietary protein should be neither too high nor too low. Bodybuilders often eat 2 grams of protein per kilogram of body weight, which is too high, as this causes elevated levels of IGF-1, a

pro-aging molecule. The Recommended Daily Allowance of protein is 0.8 gram per kilogram, which is too low, and can lead to muscle wasting and oxidative stress.

8. Practice regular intermittent fasting. At a bare minimum, do not eat snacks and do not eat between dinner and breakfast to ensure regular promotion of the anti-aging process of autophagy, which clears cellular junk and renews mitochondria. For a stronger pro-longevity effect, fast for 16 hours or more several times a week, or 24 hours once a week.

9. Finally, combine intermittent fasting, weight training, and protein feeding into a cyclical schedule, such that the natural diurnal rhythms of breakdown and renewal are reinforced. Fast for a period of time to clear cellular junk through autophagy, then train with weights (or do other forms of intense exercise) and eat sufficient protein to renew body tissues.

There's much more that I could have put into this book, since any substance or process that promotes general health and prevents illness also conduces to a longer life. But I presume that anyone interested enough in a longer life to read a book on the topic will already be doing almost all of these things, and besides, general health advice (however inaccurate or misleading) is not lacking either in books or on the internet.

The steps I've outlined in this book to slow the aging process are somewhat, but not entirely, outside of mainstream health advice. Exercise, for example, is well nigh universally recommended for better health. (Although in the mainstream, it's often assumed that more exercise is always better, and it is not.) On the other hand, fasting is still fairly outside mainstream health advise, and in fact many people think it is crazy. But it seems to be rapidly entering mainstream acceptance; in a few years time, I suspect that fasting will be as commonly touted as a healthy process as running is today.

The paleo movement has gained a lot of traction in the past few years, but mostly it is considered only under the aspect of food quality. Yet the conditions under which we evolved differ in much more than merely food: the timing of eating, the amount and types of exercise, social environment, sleep, all of these differ from the modern environment. If we want to maximize health and prolong our lives, it makes sense to pay attention to these.

However, maximizing health has only some overlap with maximizing lifespan. Aging is an entirely natural process, so in some sense we must go against nature to maximize lifespan. If reproductive capacity can be seen as a subset of health, then maximizing it also maximizes health. Yet some interventions that may increase reproductive capacity, for instance eating large amounts of protein that cause an increase in muscle mass or height in youth, may dispose towards shorter lifespan through an increase in cancer risk in later life. Calorie restriction, conversely, may decrease reproductive capacity and strength in youth while preventing disease in later life.

The scientific quest to fight aging involves the attempt to understand the nature of aging so that we can interfere with it. Until we understand how to do this, the processes outlined in this book may give us our best shot at slowing the aging process and prolonging our lives.

Bibliography

Chapter 1

1. Berbesque, J. Colette, et al. "Hunter–gatherers have less famine than agriculturalists." *Biology Letters* 10.1 (2014): 20130853.
2. Kolb, Hubert, and Décio L. Eizirik. "Resistance to type 2 diabetes mellitus: a matter of hormesis?." *Nature Reviews Endocrinology* 8.3 (2012): 183-192.
3. Radak, Zsolt, Hae Young Chung, and Sataro Goto. "Exercise and hormesis: oxidative stress-related adaptation for successful aging." *Biogerontology* 6.1 (2005): 71-75.
4. Harman, Denham. "Free radical theory of aging." *Mutation Research/DNAging* 275.3 (1992): 257-266.
5. Schmeisser, Sebastian, et al. "Mitochondrial hormesis links low-dose arsenite exposure to lifespan extension." *Aging Cell* 12.3 (2013): 508-517.
6. Franceschi, Claudio. "Inflammaging as a major characteristic of old people: can it be prevented or cured?." *Nutrition Reviews* 65.suppl 3 (2007): S173-S176.

Chapter 2: Exercise

1. Myers, Jonathan, et al. "Exercise capacity and mortality among men referred for exercise testing." *New England Journal of Medicine* 346.11 (2002): 793-801.
2. Garcia-Valles, Rebeca, et al. "Life-long spontaneous exercise does not prolong lifespan but improves health span in mice." *Longev. Healthspan* 2 (2013): 14.
3. Moore, Steven C., et al. "Leisure time physical activity of moderate to vigorous intensity and mortality: a large pooled cohort analysis." *PLoS Medicine* 9.11 (2012): e1001335.
4. Reimers, C. D., G. Knapp, and A. K. Reimers. "Does physical activity increase life expectancy? A review of the literature." *Journal of Aging Research* 2012 (2012).
5. Ruiz, Jonatan R., et al. "Muscular strength and adiposity as predictors of adulthood cancer mortality in men." *Cancer Epidemiology Biomarkers & Prevention* 18.5 (2009): 1468-1476.
6. Myers, Jonathan. "Exercise and cardiovascular health." *Circulation* 107.1 (2003): e2-e5.

7. Ristow, Michael, et al. "Antioxidants prevent health-promoting effects of physical exercise in humans." *Proceedings of the National Academy of Sciences* 106.21 (2009): 8665-8670.

8. He, Congcong, et al. "Exercise-induced BCL2-regulated autophagy is required for muscle glucose homeostasis." *Nature* 481.7382 (2012): 511-515.

8. He, Congcong, Rhea Sumpter, Jr, and Beth Levine. "Exercise induces autophagy in peripheral tissues and in the brain." *Autophagy* 8.10 (2012): 1548-1551.

9. Colcombe, Stanley J., et al. "Aerobic exercise training increases brain volume in aging humans." *The Journals of Gerontology Series A: Biological Sciences and Medical Sciences* 61.11 (2006): 1166-1170.

10. Yarrow, Joshua F., et al. "Training augments resistance exercise induced elevation of circulating brain derived neurotrophic factor (BDNF)." *Neuroscience Letters* 479.2 (2010): 161-165.

11. Faulkner, John A., et al. "Age-related changes in the structure and function of skeletal muscles." *Clinical and Experimental Pharmacology and Physiology*34.11 (2007): 1091-1096.

12. Simpson, Richard J., et al. "Exercise and the aging immune system." *Ageing Research Reviews* 11.3 (2012): 404-420.

12. Pierce, Gary L., et al. "Habitually exercising older men do not demonstrate age-associated vascular endothelial oxidative stress." *Aging Cell* 10.6 (2011): 1032-1037.

13. Schnohr, Peter, et al. "Dose of jogging and long-term mortality: the Copenhagen City Heart Study." *Journal of the American College of Cardiology* 65.5 (2015): 411-419.

14. Breuckmann, Frank, et al. "Myocardial Late Gadolinium Enhancement: Prevalence, Pattern, and Prognostic Relevance in Marathon Runners 1."*Radiology* 251.1 (2009): 50-57.

15. Wilson, Mathew, et al. "Diverse patterns of myocardial fibrosis in lifelong, veteran endurance athletes." *Journal of Applied Physiology* 110.6 (2011): 1622-1626.

16. Lowery, Lonnie, and Cassandra E. Forsythe. "Protein and overtraining: potential applications for free-living athletes." *J Int Soc Sports Nutr* 3.1 (2006): 42-50.

17. Singh, Nalin A., et al. "Effects of high-intensity progressive resistance training and targeted multidisciplinary treatment of frailty on mortality and nursing home admissions after hip fracture: a randomized controlled trial." *Journal of the American Medical Directors Association* 13.1 (2012): 24-30.

18. Boutcher, Stephen H. "High-intensity intermittent exercise and fat loss."*Journal of Obesity* 2011 (2010).

19. Little, Jonathan P., et al. "A practical model of low-volume high-intensity interval training induces mitochondrial biogenesis in human skeletal muscle: potential mechanisms." *The Journal of Physiology* 588.6 (2010): 1011-1022.
20. Ortega, J. F., et al. "Higher Insulin-sensitizing Response after Sprint Interval Compared to Continuous Exercise." *International Journal of Sports Medicine*(2014).

Chapter 3: Diet

1. Bigaard, Janne, et al. "Body fat and fat-free mass and all-cause mortality."*Obesity Research* 12.7 (2004): 1042-1049.
2. Stokes, Andrew. "Using maximum weight to redefine body mass index categories in studies of the mortality risks of obesity." *Population Health Metrics* 12.1 (2014): 6. Fontana, Luigi, and Frank B. Hu. "Optimal body weight for health and longevity: bridging basic, clinical, and population research." *Aging Cell* 13.3 (2014): 391-400.
3. Kenyon, Cynthia, et al. "A C. elegans mutant that lives twice as long as wild type." *Nature* 366.6454 (1993): 461-464.
4. The Guardian, 16 March 2013
5. Lee, Seung-Jae, Coleen T. Murphy, and Cynthia Kenyon. "Glucose shortens the life span of C. elegans by downregulating DAF-16/FOXO activity and aquaporin gene expression." *Cell Metabolism* 10.5 (2009): 379-391.
6. Schulz, Tim J., et al. "Glucose restriction extends Caenorhabditis elegans life span by inducing mitochondrial respiration and increasing oxidative stress."*Cell Metabolism* 6.4 (2007): 280-293.
7. Tatar, Marc, Andrzej Bartke, and Adam Antebi. "The endocrine regulation of aging by insulin-like signals." *Science* 299.5611 (2003): 1346-1351.
8. Kurosu, Hiroshi, et al. "Suppression of aging in mice by the hormone Klotho."*Science* 309.5742 (2005): 1829-1833.
9. Lindeberg, Staffan, et al. "Low serum insulin in traditional Pacific Islanders—the Kitava Study." *Metabolism* 48.10 (1999): 1216-1219.
10. Rosedale, Ron, Eric C. Westman, and John P. Konhilas. "Clinical experience of a diet designed to reduce aging." *The Journal of Applied Research* 9.4 (2009): 159.
11. Klement, Rainer J., and Ulrike Kämmerer. "Is there a role for carbohydrate restriction in the treatment and prevention of cancer." *Nutr Metab (Lond)* 8.75 (2011): 75.

12. Accurso, Anthony, et al. "Dietary carbohydrate restriction in type 2 diabetes mellitus and metabolic syndrome: time for a critical appraisal." *Nutrition & Metabolism* 5.1 (2008): 9.

13. Klein, S., and R R. Wolfe. "Carbohydrate restriction regulates the adaptive response to fasting." *American Journal of Physiology-Endocrinology and Metabolism* 262.5 (1992): E631-E636.

14. Salminen, Antero, and Kai Kaarniranta. "AMP-activated protein kinase (AMPK) controls the aging process via an integrated signaling network." *Ageing Research Reviews* 11.2 (2012): 230-241.

15. Baur, Joseph A., et al. "Resveratrol improves health and survival of mice on a high-calorie diet." *Nature* 444.7117 (2006): 337-342.

16. Witte, A. Veronica, et al. "Effects of resveratrol on memory performance, hippocampal functional connectivity, and glucose metabolism in healthy older adults." *The Journal of Neuroscience* 34.23 (2014): 7862-7870.

17. Timmers, Silvie, et al. "Calorie restriction-like effects of 30 days of resveratrol supplementation on energy metabolism and metabolic profile in obese humans." *Cell Metabolism* 14.5 (2011): 612-622.

18. Hsu, Shih-Che, et al. "Resveratrol increases anti-aging Klotho gene expression via the activating transcription factor 3/c-Jun complex-mediated signaling pathway." *The International Journal of Biochemistry & Cell Biology* 53 (2014): 361-371.

19. Jang, Meishiang, et al. "Cancer chemopreventive activity of resveratrol, a natural product derived from grapes." *Science* 275.5297 (1997): 218-220.

20. Russo, Maria, et al. "The flavonoid quercetin in disease prevention and therapy: facts and fancies." *Biochemical pharmacology* 83.1 (2012): 6-15.

21. Zhu, Yi et al., The Achilles' Heel of Senescent Cells: From Transcriptome to Senolytic Drugs, *Aging Cell*, DOI: 10.1111/acel.12344

22. Pietrocola, Federico, et al. "Coffee induces autophagy in vivo." *Cell Cycle* 13.12 (2014): 1987-1994.

23. Kitani, Kenichi, Toshihiko Osawa, and Takako Yokozawa. "The effects of tetrahydrocurcumin and green tea polyphenol on the survival of male C57BL/6 mice." *Biogerontology* 8.5 (2007): 567-573.

24. Niu, Yucun, et al. "The phytochemical, EGCG, extends lifespan by reducing liver and kidney function damage and improving age-associated inflammation and oxidative stress in healthy rats." *Aging Cell* 12.6 (2013): 1041-1049.

25. Zarse, Kim, et al. "Low-dose lithium uptake promotes longevity in humans and metazoans." *European Journal of Nutrition* 50.5 (2011): 387-389.

26. Wan, Qin-Li, et al. "Aspirin extends the lifespan of Caenorhabditis elegans via AMPK and DAF-16/FOXO in dietary restriction pathway." *Experimental Gerontology* 48.5 (2013): 499-506.

27. Guevara-Aguirre, Jaime, et al. "Growth hormone receptor deficiency is associated with a major reduction in pro-aging signaling, cancer, and diabetes in humans." *Science Translational Medicine* 3.70 (2011): 70ra13-70ra13.

28. Richie, JOHN P., et al. "Methionine restriction increases blood glutathione and longevity in F344 rats." *The FASEB Journal* 8.15 (1994): 1302-1307.

29. Fontana, Luigi, et al. "Long-term effects of calorie or protein restriction on serum IGF-1 and IGFBP-3 concentration in humans." *Aging Cell* 7.5 (2008): 681-687.

30. Tarnopolsky, M. A., et al. "Evaluation of protein requirements for trained strength athletes." *Journal of Applied Physiology* 73.5 (1992): 1986-1995.

31. Walker, KYLIE S., et al. "Resistance training alters plasma myostatin but not IGF-1 in healthy men." *Medicine and Science in Sports and Exercise* 36.5 (2004): 787-793.

32. Wolfe, Robert R. "The underappreciated role of muscle in health and disease."*The American Journal of Clinical Nutrition* 84.3 (2006): 475-482.

33. Mirzaei, Hamed, Jorge A. Suarez, and Valter D. Longo. "Protein and amino acid restriction, aging and disease: from yeast to humans." *Trends in Endocrinology & Metabolism* 25.11 (2014): 558-566.

Chapter 4: Fasting

1. Cornaro, A, Discourses on the temperate life. http://www.soilandhealth.org/02/0201hyglibcat/020105c ornaro.html

2. Goldberg, Emily L., et al. "Lifespan-extending caloric restriction or mTOR inhibition impair adaptive immunity of old mice by distinct mechanisms." *Aging Cell* (2014).

3. Anson, R. Michael, et al. "Intermittent fasting dissociates beneficial effects of dietary restriction on glucose metabolism and

neuronal resistance to injury from calorie intake." *Proceedings of the National Academy of Sciences* 100.10 (2003): 6216-6220.

4. Mattson, Mark P., and Ruiqian Wan. "Beneficial effects of intermittent fasting and caloric restriction on the cardiovascular and cerebrovascular systems."*The Journal of Nutritional Biochemistry* 16.3 (2005): 129-137.

5. Reardon, Michael, and Marek Malik. "Changes in heart rate variability with age." *Pacing and Clinical Electrophysiology* 19.11 (1996): 1863-1866.

6. Martin, Bronwen, Mark P. Mattson, and Stuart Maudsley. "Caloric restriction and intermittent fasting: two potential diets for successful brain aging." *Ageing Research Reviews* 5.3 (2006): 332-353.

7. Tajes, M., et al. "Neuroprotective role of intermittent fasting in senescence-accelerated mice P8 (SAMP8)." *Experimental Gerontology* 45.9 (2010): 702-710.

8. Katare, Rajesh G., et al. "Chronic intermittent fasting improves the survival following large myocardial ischemia by activation of BDNF/VEGF/PI3K signaling pathway." *Journal of Molecular and Cellular Cardiology* 46.3 (2009): 405-412.

9. Alirezaei, Mehrdad, et al. "Short-term fasting induces profound neuronal autophagy." *Autophagy* 6.6 (2010): 702-710.

10. IGF-1 & Intermittent Fasting: Discussion with Valter Longo. http://michelsonmedical.org/2014/12/26/igf-1-fasting-discussion-valter-longo/

11. Safdie, Fernando M., et al. "Fasting and cancer treatment in humans: A case series report." *Aging (Albany NY)* 1.12 (2009): 988.

12. Cheng, Chia-Wei, et al. "Prolonged fasting reduces IGF-1/PKA to promote hematopoietic-stem-cell-based regeneration and reverse immunosuppression."*Cell Stem Cell* 14.6 (2014): 810-823.

13. Moore, Jimmy. "Seyfried Cancer Textbook Cites My 7-Day Fast Experience." http://livinlavidalowcarb.com/blog/seyfried-cancer-textbook-cites-my-7-day-fast-experience/14541

14. Mariño, Guillermo, et al. "Caloric restriction mimetics: natural/physiological pharmacological autophagy inducers." *Autophagy* 10.11 (2014): 1879-1882.

15. Mattson, Mark P. "Challenging Oneself Intermittently to Improve Health." *Dose-Response* 12.4 (2014): 600.

Chapter 5: Demolition and Renewal

1. Cuervo, Ana Maria, et al. "Autophagy and aging: the importance of maintaining "clean" cells." *Autophagy* 1.3 (2005): 131-140.

2. Bratic, Ana, and Nils-Göran Larsson. "The role of mitochondria in aging." *The Journal of clinical investigation* 123.123 (3) (2013): 951-957.

3. Ristow, Michael, et al. "Antioxidants prevent health-promoting effects of physical exercise in humans." *Proceedings of the National Academy of Sciences* 106.21 (2009): 8665-8670.

4. Dröge, Wulf. "Oxidative stress and ageing: is ageing a cysteine deficiency syndrome?." *Philosophical Transactions of the Royal Society B: Biological Sciences* 360.1464 (2005): 2355-2372.

5. Sekhar, Rajagopal V., et al. "Deficient synthesis of glutathione underlies oxidative stress in aging and can be corrected by dietary cysteine and glycine supplementation." *The American Journal of Clinical Nutrition* 94.3 (2011): 847-853. \

6. Kent, K. D., W. J. Harper, and J. A. Bomser. "Effect of whey protein isolate on intracellular glutathione and oxidant-induced cell death in human prostate epithelial cells." *Toxicology in vitro* 17.1 (2003): 27-33.

7. Sekhar, Rajagopal V., et al. "Deficient synthesis of glutathione underlies oxidative stress in aging and can be corrected by dietary cysteine and glycine supplementation." *The American Journal of Clinical Nutrition* 94.3 (2011): 847-853.

8. Chen, Chiao-nan Joyce, et al. "Late-onset Caloric Restriction Alters Skeletal Muscle Metabolism by Modulating Pyruvate Metabolism." *American Journal of Physiology-Endocrinology and Metabolism* (2015): ajpendo-00508.

9. Ho, Klan Y., et al. "Fasting enhances growth hormone secretion and amplifies the complex rhythms of growth hormone secretion in man." *Journal of Clinical Investigation* 81.4 (1988): 968.

10. Hoffman, Jay R., and Michael J. Falvo. "Protein—which is best?." *Journal of Sports Science & Medicine* 3.3 (2004): 118.

11. Tarnopolsky, Mark A., J. Duncan MacDougall, and Stephanie A. Atkinson. "Influence of protein intake and training status on nitrogen balance and lean body mass." *Journal of Applied Physiology* 64.1 (1988): 187-193.

About the author

P. D. Mangan has written a number of books on health and fitness, of which this is his fourth. The others include Smash Chronic Fatigue, Best Supplements for Men's Health, Strength, and Virility, and Top Ten reasons We're Fat. They can all be found on his Amazon Author page. He blogs at Rogue Health and Fitness.com.

Made in the USA
Columbia, SC
12 January 2018